AM I NORMAL?

Understanding your place in a complex world

DR ALEX GEORGE

ASTER*

First published in Great Britain in 2026 by Aster, an imprint of

Octopus Publishing Group Ltd
Carmelite House
50 Victoria Embankment
London EC4Y 0DZ
www.octopusbooks.co.uk

An Hachette UK Company
www.hachette.co.uk

The authorised representative in the EEA is Hachette Ireland,
8 Castlecourt Centre, Dublin 15, D15 XTP3, Ireland (email: info@hbgi.ie)

Text Copyright © Dr Alex George 2026
Copyright © Octopus Publishing Group Ltd 2026

Distributed in the US by
Hachette Book Group
1290 Avenue of the Americas
4th and 5th Floors
New York, NY 10104

Distributed in Canada by
Canadian Manda Group
664 Annette St
Toronto, Ontario, Canada M6S 2C8

ISBN (Hardback): 978-1-78325-638-9
ISBN (Trade Paperback): 978-1-78325-639-6
eISBN: 978-1-78325-495-8

A CIP catalogue record for this book is available from the British Library.

Typeset in 12.25/20pt Heldane Text by Six Red Marbles UK, Thetford, Norfolk

Printed and bound in Great Britain.

10 9 8 7 6 5 4 3 2

Commissioning Editor: Katie Forsythe
Senior Editor: Alex Stetter
Creative Director: Mel Four
Senior Production Manager: Peter Hunt

Additional picture credit: page 4, Andrii Ablohin/iStock

This FSC® label means that materials used for the product have been responsibly sourced.

AM I NORMAL?

I dedicate this book to Mam and Dad.

I love you ever so much.

CONTENTS

INTRODUCTION

To a doctor, 'normal' means healthy and it means right. For a long time, I thought that if I had a normal job, a normal social life and even a normal experience of grief, my life would progress without too much friction or pain. I believed that although I might *be* different, if I could just live as everyone else seemed to, I would feel alright.

So imagine my surprise when these attempts to live normally began to make me sick. My normal job (doctor) and my normal way of approaching it (relentlessly) were burning me out. My 'normal' social life was dragging me down a path to alcohol misuse and the secret, private form of grief that I suffered in the name of normality had pulled me into the depths of a deep depression.

I was stuck. I couldn't continue on the path I was on. I was the heaviest I had ever been, drinking more than I ever had and suffering because the sharp edges of my grief would not soften with time or self-medication. I knew I had to change – but how?

How could I find that 'normal function' that doctors speak of in my personal, professional and social lives? How could I move through the world if the struggle to be normal was the very thing that was causing me distress?

The seed of a revelation took root in a barber's chair, that awkward place where we are confronted with a reflection of ourselves that we have tried to avoid. On that day, I looked at myself in the mirror and saw a man at breaking point. My face and my body showed signs of the pain that I thought I had hidden. The suffering that I believed to be silent screamed out from my sunken eyes, my drooping shoulders and my greying skin.

It began to dawn on me that my suffering was in part my own creation. The loss of my brother, my life-long anxiety and tendency to excess were not my choice, but the decision to hide them in the name of keeping up appearances was, and it became clear that this was the first thing I needed to change. I could no longer keep pulling myself out of shape in the name of fitting in. I could not keep living my life by a set of norms that I had never interrogated and accepting unhappiness as a result of trying to fit within them. Up to that point, I had really never stopped to question the norms that I lived by, the self that was struggling with them or the assumption that it was better to suffer normally than flourish on my own terms. No more.

By the time the barber pulled his cape from across my shoulders, I was reignited with a purpose – not healed or cured, but finally motivated by something approaching a plan of action. I knew something had to change: I had no other choice. I would tackle my discomfort from two directions: by understanding the society I tried to fit into and the self that I had constantly stretched out of shape to do so.

First, I had to try to understand what it is that we call normal. In our schools, workplaces and weekends, we all seem to agree on certain ways of doing things without ever interrogating why this is the case. So I began to question them. Why is a child who can sit at a desk for an hour normal but the one who wants to move and explore the world in a different way abnormal? Why do we celebrate *and* commiserate with alcohol and feel like the odd one out when we choose not to drink? Why do we feel so weird talking about death when we know it's a part of everyone's human experience?

These ways of being, and of doing, are not a result of our nature but our cultures, and it is only because we repeat them so often that they don't ever seem strange to us. They are norms that have been chosen, prioritised and encouraged. In some cases, they have remained in place because they allow for a certain uniformity and simplicity, and in others because certain industries (alcohol, tech, food) benefit from them. Most of all, however, I think our norms endure because most of us haven't had the opportunity or space to question their utility.

My hope is that this book will encourage a conversation about who we build our society for, who we include and who we let down, because norms dictate individual lives but they also drive policy and the shape of society itself. In some instances, what we consider normal might be working quite well for everyone. In others, it may suit the majority in the middle but leave those on the edges struggling and forgotten, outliers to fall through the cracks.

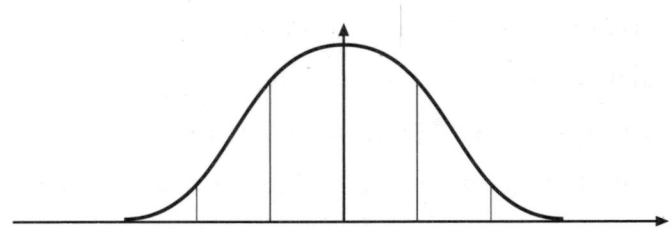

In a bell curve, the average (or 'normal') value is also the most common.

It can be useful to think about a bell curve here. You've probably seen one before. It's a graph that looks like a bell, with a peak around the middle and a decline out towards the edges.

The bell curve describes the distribution of points – in this context, people – across a set – here, society. What this shape shows is what we could describe 'normal' as the very middle of that graph because that is the point where there is the largest group of similar people. Everyone at the edges of the bell shape are the 'outliers', whom we might consider to be 'different'. These outliers, in the context of our society's norms, are those who, for reasons of trauma, neurodiversity or disability, do not fit into the system and who are then framed as problems or left to languish outside of the scope of society's provisions.

This book looks at my life and the norms that have shaped it. My intention is to use my own experience to better understand where norms have helped and where they have hindered. In those cases where it seems that norms have made me, and others, unhappy or unhealthy, I will suggest alternative ways of moving through the world which could allow myself and others to live authentically. Do not worry, though, if you like doing things the 'normal way'. This is not to say that we should limit anyone's freedom to behave as they always have done, just that we open up room for a greater range of people to flourish in their unique ways.

If you have ever struggled and wondered (quite normally) 'Am I normal?', then this book is for you. It is an opportunity for me to show that other ways of doing things are possible and that it may be better to try to change aspects of our society before we labour to remake ourselves. In many cases, the shape of this new culture and its norms will follow the shape of our diversity as humans. Some things that are currently thought of as strange should, in my eyes, be considered normal. Some things that are the norm should really be considered exceptions to the rule.

So here are some ways in which I am normal, and I am not:

I am not normal because I have chosen to speak publicly about suicide and grief. The normal response to grief, as governed by (British) social norms, is to be quiet about it and in the context of suicide, to be silent. In this case, speaking up and showing vulnerability is abnormal, but it is also crucial if we are to create healthier norms around grief. Therefore, my abnormality is a necessary price to pay for the normalisation of something important. Again, this reflects how normal does not mean right and how abnormality is something to strive for when we want to make a change.

I am normal because I have had problematic relationships with food, alcohol and digital media, and abnormal because I am unashamed to discuss it. These very normal things can be harmful and addictive, and the way our society presents and regulates them is problematic. The question we must ask is why we allow our very normal potential for addiction to be turned into profit models and become cornerstones of our society. I am abnormal for pointing that out, and I am proud. Most of all, I am abnormal because I am not afraid to admit that I am. The most pernicious thing about our culture of normality is the pain that is created when we try to mask our differences. The greatest suffering comes when we try to contort ourselves into shapes to fit the boxes that our culture designs.

It should be normal not to be normal. It should be one of the great aims of a progressive society to expand its reach to include its outliers. The bell curve should not feel like a mountain to climb for those who sit at its edges because our difference should not cause isolation. It is not for sentimental reasons or inclusivity for inclusion's sake that I say this. Understanding and valuing differences is not only about how people feel but how our society succeeds. In fact, we can chart the progress of history by looking at the gradually broadening scope of who 'counts' in society. For example, education went from serving elite males to include those from the middle classes, before accepting women and those from working-class backgrounds. From my experience, we still struggle to adequately serve those who are neurodiverse or have suffered trauma, and this represents the next step of our progress.

If we increase the scope of who counts, who fits into our norms in spaces like education, we could save many people from isolation and loneliness, and save society from the harms and costs that will inevitably present later on in its healthcare and justice systems. We move forward by casting our net wider.

So in the name of a more inclusive and better-functioning society, I will tell you my story. It is the story of my difference, of the schools where I was considered incapable because I thought and learned differently to others. Of my unexpected success in an A&E department, where an abnormal brain is actually quite a useful one. It will be a discussion of the ways I was told to be. I hope that reading it will help you to grow in your understanding of yourself, to see the ways in which your differences can be your strengths and to realise that the suffering that comes with difference is not the result of your failings. This book aims to be a call to action. Sometimes, our pain is an alarm that tells us that something in our world needs to change.

I also hope you'll gain greater empathy for those who have been let down by a society that cannot account for their differences. Our prisons are home to many individuals who, because of trauma, brain chemistry or difficult home environments, behaved and presented in ways that saw them problematised in childhood. Our healthcare system is full of people who grew sick because of the 'normal' ways of eating, drinking and living that have been encouraged for years. Our morgues are full of young men who took their own lives because they lived in a society that told them not to speak about their feelings.

I may not be normal. Maybe none of us are. But we have the ability to create a more considered and inclusive society that normalises the things that make us happier and healthier, and allows people to be happy and healthy even when they are different. I hope my small journey sheds some light on what change could look like.

My story is sometimes sad but it is often hilarious. It's unique, of course, but defined by moments of connection and community that remind us what it is to be human, to feel that we belong. It is odd, rich and human, and, as strange as it may make me seem, as abnormal as it may make me, I am not ashamed to tell it.

This is the story of all of the ways in which I didn't fit in and of all the things I would rather change in the world than myself.

PROLOGUE: THE PSYCHIATRIST'S OFFICE

Some time after I sat in a barber's chair and accepted that I might not be normal, I waited in another chair for a psychiatrist to tell me how. I had been diagnosed with attention deficit hyperactivity disorder (ADHD), depression and the sort of grief that needs something more than the passing thoughts and prayers of acquaintances. I felt broken, but grateful for the simple fact that I knew it. The only thing worse than seeing the shattered pieces of yourself, is failing to recognise them.

I was one step closer to picking up those pieces and to finding something adhesive in my life that could bring them back together. What I would build, I would build on my terms, starting from an understanding of myself rather than the desire to fit with what was expected of me.

So that is where we began. My psychiatrist asked me some questions that drove at the heart of who I was and who I had been, rather than whoever I thought I should be. No longer was the starting point what I needed to do, but how I felt, how I had experienced the world and how I could move through it without fear or friction. This meant looking at my past and present before charting the course of my future. We had to discuss what my childhood was like, what made me feel alone and what gave me comfort. We had to look back at my work, identify the places where I experienced belonging and the reasons I had often felt so alone. We had to talk about love, loss and friendship, the life I had led and the bereavement that almost consumed me.

I had to answer my doctor's questions but in reality, I had to answer to myself. I may not have been responsible for all the hardships that shaped me, but I was responsible for learning their lessons and breaking the cycles of a lifetime that made me unhappy. I had to accept myself – and to do so, I had to understand myself.

So together, that's what we did, and now those questions form the basis of this book. Each chapter grows from one of them, from the evaluation of my experience to the discussion of my difference, through to the revelation that difference is not in itself a problem. The problem is a world that makes no room for difference. The solution I found was seeing that while many things in our lives can be changed, some things about ourselves should not be, if changing them causes us distress. In these cases, the question is not whether our difference makes us *wrong* but what is so right about the norm from which we deviate?

So I want to do that with you. To tell you about my answers to the questions a psychiatrist asked, the discoveries I made of my oddities and the clarity I feel in my belief that being abnormal is just about the most normal thing we can be. Then I want to think about how we can create a society that flourishes in acceptance of that. Which grounds, to some extent, my answer to her first question.

Why are you here?

1

WHY ARE YOU HERE?

Like many moments of self-discovery, mine came in a field, listening to a house DJ. He didn't play any music and it really wasn't the right moment to dance. Instead, he told me about his recent ADHD diagnosis and experience of sobriety, and something within me clicked. I believe this is what raving becomes in your thirties. That DJ was Toddla T, and in September 2022 he was a guest on my podcast, the Stompcast, which I record outdoors. During the interview, Toddla T described how he came to understand years of impulsive behaviour, organisational challenges and issues around alcohol through his ADHD diagnosis. He told me it had changed his life and, in the process, he changed mine too.

It's funny to listen back to that interview now. You can hear that I am struggling to be professional while having a massive personal revelation, which isn't an easy thing to do. As an interviewer, your focus should be on your guest as you try to delve into their experiences and probe them on their motivations. You should *not* glaze over and repeatedly think, *Gosh! He's talking about me!* I do not recommend this as an approach to broadcasting or an initial assessment for neurodiversity, but I have to admit it helped me. My conversation with Toddla T led me to organise my own assessment for ADHD, a neurodevelopmental condition that can manifest in many ways but is classically defined through challenges with impulsivity, attention and hyperactivity – or at least, challenges with regulating those things in a 'normal' way.

The irony of coming to the conclusion that I may have ADHD symptoms while failing to pay proper attention to someone as we both walked very quickly (hyperactively, even) around a green space is not lost on me. Irony is something I have grown comfortable with as an ADHDer. Many of my current behaviours and past actions come into sharp and often ironic focus with the benefit of my diagnosis. I am a socially anxious person who accidentally became a public figure. My neurodevelopmental condition is a large part of how I became an A&E doctor. I'm writing a book about my life because I have so often struggled to evaluate my past in a healthy way. Maybe normal lives are not ironic but I've learned to see these ironies as adding colour to my experience.

Evaluating my experiences became a key component of making progress once I decided to get an ADHD assessment. I had considered getting myself assessed for it in the past, but the process seemed daunting and involved too many components for my poorly organised and often anxious mind. (Here we see irony again: my ADHD holding me back from discovering that I had it.)

But Toddla T had planted a seed and this time I was prepared to navigate any complexity to see what might grow from it. So I organised a call with a psychiatrist who would evaluate me, safe in the knowledge that this time I would go through with it, even though it filled me with dread.

Even though I knew I needed to sort my life out, because I was in a bad way, struggling with self-destructive behaviours and poor mental health, I still had my doubts. I worried that any abnormality I felt was a figment of my imagination, that the psychiatrist would think I was wasting her time with nothing more than projection of my own anxiety. Why did it take a Stompcast recording with a DJ to recognise that something might be amiss, that perhaps I was not normal? Should I not have been able to recognise myself, especially as a doctor?

So I was certain that when she asked 'why are you here?', it would be laden with criticism, rather than the open and empathetic call to share that it really was. When the day of the assessment came, I knew what my answer to that question was, even though I felt afraid to admit it. I was there because I wanted to understand myself – why I felt and acted the way that I did, and whether it was normal. I couldn't blame the world for the self-destructive pattern that I was in, drinking, struggling with rapid weight gain and intrusive thoughts, but I suspected that if I understood more, I wouldn't just blame myself either. There had to be some information about myself or the world that explained why it all felt so uncomfortable.

Unsurprisingly, the psychiatrist was kind and professional. We began the assessment by addressing questions that would help draw the picture of my life. I completed the questions before we spoke and I recall experiencing a similar feeling to the one I had during my conversation with Toddla T. I felt as if the person who had written them on that sheet of A4 had some secret insight into my own life, a hidden camera or network of spies, that allowed them to understand my experiences in ways that even I struggled to do.

Do you feel compelled to do things like you were driven by a motor?
Yes, a V8 engine specifically. The horsepower is incredible but some work is needed on the torque and brakes. Oh, and it breaks down on the roadside often.

How often do you interrupt others when—?
Yes!

You see, each question felt more like a description of my life than a generic diagnostic criterion, and that gave me a sense of what the outcome was going to be before I had even finished. My friend Adam, who I put forward as a second interviewee, said the same. If I didn't have ADHD, then it was quite the coincidence that I matched so well with its symptoms.

When you have an assessment, you're asked to provide one or two family members or friends who can offer their own description of aspects of your life and personality. This allows the psychiatrist to get a broader picture of your behaviour and accounts for the fact that many of us remember our lives and experiences in different ways. My parents, for example, answered the questions very differently to me and Adam. When they shared their answers with me, I was frustrated and angry. I believed that they were trying to will me into normality with wishful thinking and a rose-tinted view of my past, but with time, I have understood their account. It's real for them, and no two people see any one thing in the same way. Someone can see their own past in entirely different ways depending on the moment they are in and the perspectives they can access. My life story would be a very different one if I were telling it two years ago; my history would be written differently if I were less comfortable in myself than I am now. This book is my response to that fact.

I may be comfortable now but as the psychiatrist opened my questionnaire to discuss the questions I had answered and add a few of her own, I was terrified. I didn't see a pathway towards self-knowledge awaiting me so much as a deep pit of damning criticism. As I saw it, another doctor was about to confirm that the way I felt was the way I appeared to the world: abnormal and broken beyond repair. My private shame was about to become public.

You will be glad to know that this was only partly true. I was broken and I wasn't normal, but I wasn't beyond repair, and it was only by understanding my difference and my pain that I was going to feel better. The problem wasn't that I was abnormal, but that I had decided it was easier to suffer than acknowledge it.

The psychiatrist began to discuss my answers and relief set in. There was no shame and no criticism, no 'gotcha' moment where I was unmasked and shown to be less worthwhile. A lifelong fear of being different became a reality and I started to feel . . . better. Somehow, it made me feel less alone, as if difference itself was not the problem but the belief that it would mean I was beyond help. I was a square peg being told that the world could contain more than just round holes.

Each step of her diagnosis gave me a framework for understanding my function, reasons to reevaluate my experience and tools to approach my future. I am telling my life story because I have reappraised it in recent years, and I am beginning that story with my ADHD diagnosis because it is the very thing that has allowed me to do it. Everything, from my childhood to my work and relationships, came into sharper focus with the clarity that my diagnosis provided. I understand how and why I behaved in the way that I did, and that my problem didn't have to be *such a problem* if society broadened its scope of understanding. My brain wasn't 'normal' but I didn't have to suffer because of it.

The main point of difference in an ADHD mind is its 'executive function': just imagine my brain were a business, with quite an erratic chief executive. This presents as an inability to manage our present behaviour so that demands for the future can be met. The part of my brain that considers where I have been, where I want to go and how to move successfully between them can be disjointed. This can result in issues with getting easily distracted, but it can also feed into impulsive behaviour (like buying motorbikes before being able to ride them or making spur-of-the-moment decisions to go on reality television) and a difficulty with self-talk (the conversations we all have, with ourselves, in our own minds). Overthinking and difficulty with managing thoughts is common in ADHD, as are issues with emotional regulation. The pre-frontal cortex helps manage the way we react to life as well as the thoughts in our heads.

I have always struggled with the way I talk to myself, being my own worst critic to a ridiculous extent. This can have a ruminative and cyclical feel and pattern. The inability to put on the brakes, as it were, means that you can really get in a rut.

No two people with ADHD are the same, though, (there is no normal here!) and, as you will see, many aspects of my condition are quite particular to me, while others fit more general patterns. Before my diagnosis, I thought about these things only in terms of my personality, which they also are. I thought I was a hedonist, a person who lived in the now, who decided they wanted to ride a motorbike and booked the test and started shopping for bikes the same day. When I went for a beer, I went for one and then left having had far more. I soon realised these things weren't hedonistic but a lack of executive function at play.

It is with self-talk that I have some more personal challenges. Often, people with ADHD are considered to have a limited capacity for self-talk, which means that while we may have an angel and a devil on each shoulder, we struggle to manage the debate between the two. Lacking this dialogue is sometimes put forward as a reason why people with ADHD don't make brilliant connections between past experiences, present behaviours and future goals. If you don't weigh up the case of the angel who reminds you of how something made you feel in the past and the devil who tells you how good something might make you feel now, it can be hard to strike a balance between the two.

This is not the case for me, as I actually have quite a pronounced sense of self-talk. Like many people with ADHD, I live in the present, but in my case, it is overloaded with negative awareness of past experiences (rumination) and focus on future doubts (anxiety). People talk about the 'four-second rule' for ADHD, which describes making decisions based on how we are feeling within a four-second span. This is not always true but in my case it largely is, with the key difference that my present, my 'four seconds', can be laden with the weight of both past and future, and therefore feel unmanageable. The present often ends up unenjoyable and the past rarely gets processed effectively, so I get stuck in endless circles of rumination without any clear end point. It was only by understanding my mind and working to break out of these four-second loops of rumination that I have begun to make my present enjoyable and my past understandable.

This example is yet another reminder of how our view can be obscured by an idea of normality. Even my neurodivergence veers from the pattern of thinking that we associate with ADHD minds, so we should always be prepared for the unique and different ways that brains work. Your mind, whether it's neurotypical or not, will differ from others in unique ways, and the more you can understand it and how it relates to the world around you, the happier and more comfortable you will be in your difference.

It's funny how different people can be. I recently spoke with two of my colleagues about self-talk and the idea of an internal monologue (or dialogue, at times). I was surprised to find out that they don't really have one. I had been led to believe that everyone was engaging in constant self-chat, yet it seems that my ADHD combined with my anxiety means that I may just speak to myself far more than many other people do. With understanding and support, this doesn't have to be a problem; difference can provide unique perspective and capabilities if we understand it and facilitate it. Although the term ADHD refers to attention *deficit* hyperactivity disorder, I don't necessarily see it that way. In fact, I think any deficit we see is more of a tension that arises when ADHD minds are forced into the expectations of a neurotypical society. In the right contexts, ADHDers are creative, resourceful and driven people who can engage in deep focus and energetic pursuit of goals – we may just approach those goals differently.

So I take issue with the idea of ADHDers having an attention *deficit* and instead prefer to think of us as having an attention *difference.* It's only because we think of normal attention spans as proper (and superior) that we can say something different is a deficit. In fact, many ADHDers I know have something more like an attention surplus, but with different ways of stimulating that attention and holding it. This illustrates one of the challenges that ideas about normality presents. If we start with an idea of 'normal' that is based on the frequency of a disposition (that is to say, 'normal' means 'most common'), and then allow the word to morph and instead refer to value ('normal' means 'correct'), we end up seeing a difference as a deficit or an excess. The word 'normal' loses its proper meaning and outliers get cast as problems or inadequacies. A difference becomes a deficit.

There's an account of the ADHD mind that I find illustrative, if not necessarily scientific, in how it shows people's differences rather than their deficits. It imagines us as hunters in a farmer's world.

Our constant awareness of external stimuli ('lack' of attention), deep focus on only the most interesting tasks and high-energy levels ('hyperactivity') are perfect for the requirements of a hunter but often don't sit comfortably with what we ask of most people in a modern society. Instead of hunters, we ask for farmers. This requires the ability to manage numerous (sometimes mundane) tasks, to organise and maintain, and to work for long periods on projects that may not necessarily engage or interest us in the short term. We are told to ignore the rabbits running past and to focus on growing things over seasons rather than catching whatever presents itself now.

This is where hyperactivity comes in. Again, I think the idea of hyperactivity often only refers to a deviation from a norm – a norm that can be questioned. We have normalised sedentary lifestyles. In fact, we have gone far beyond a farmer's world to a bureaucratic one, which is far less active than any hunter or farmer would be used to. To most people throughout human history, based on their norms, modern humans would look like we suffer from some kind of hyper-sedentary disorder. Their norm would involve many thousands of steps a day, some running and jumping, maybe the odd bit of hunting. To them, the image of a person sitting on a chair for nine hours, then switching to a moving chair (car) and a bigger chair (sofa) before going to bed, would look problematic: it would be abnormal.

This is not to say that a strong desire for physical activity is somehow better than a disposition that lends itself to office work, but rather that that neither one of them should be *normal* in the value sense. It's not better to be either a hunter, a farmer or an office worker. A person who could sit down and focus all day might have been considered defective by the hunter-gathering Saan people in Botswana or among farmers in West Wales a century ago, while kids who would rather chase squirrels than sit quietly are treated as if they are abnormal now. What society asks of us, and therefore deems normal, has changed over time.

Our society asks us to organise the world and keep it in order, and those who don't or can't subscribe to this norm are considered to have a disorder. We ask children to be planners, organisers and memorisers, and so it is no surprise that education can be such a challenge for people like me, whose attention spans don't fit into the 'normal' framework. Managing, ordering and organising are not my strong suits. If you give me one big project to plan over six months, ask me to create a timeline and deliver it on schedule, I will struggle. Frankly, I will probably fail. Whereas if you throw me into a crisis, where challenges are emerging rapidly and fires need to be put out urgently, I will not only flourish, I will probably enjoy myself. I have to approach organisation in a way that fits with my event horizon, that separates projects into broad, long-term aims and immediate tasks. With this separation I can flourish, and I'm lucky enough to work with a team who understand how to make that happen. By understanding the ways in which my brain works best and helping others to work with me in that way, I can do my best work and (hopefully) not cause my colleagues too much stress in the process.

This cycle of awareness, adaptation and development is

something that we can all use to achieve a more comfortable relationship between the nature of our minds and the demands of our
world. I framed my project of self-understanding through the lens
of ADHD, but we could all benefit from a better understanding of
our unique way of thinking. It does, however, take work and time.

I received a diagnosis straight after my assessment, and I
was very grateful for that, as my tendency to overthink would
have made any wait unbearable. The psychiatrist explained
that my first step would be to evaluate the behaviours that were
both driving and being driven by my ADHD, and to adopt new
lifestyle approaches that would allow me to flourish. I took some
time before I began taking those steps and for a few months I
kept drinking, overthinking and overworking as if nothing had
changed at all.

Soon, though, the psychiatrist's advice filtered through. I knew
that there were reasons I was acting in the way I was, and approaches
existed that could make me more resilient, better informed and
fundamentally happier. So, after a few months of evaluation and
gradual progress, I returned to my psychiatrist and told her that I
was taking the first step, the key step: stopping drinking. Drinking
alcohol is both an impulsive behaviour and a cause of impulsiveness
itself. At first, it felt like it would be impossible to avoid because it
was a significant presence in my life and society at large, but I knew
I had to try.

I had used alcohol for many years as a form of anxiety medication,
a social lubricant and a crux, but I knew by this point it was much
more a cause of my problems than a solution. My psychiatrist agreed

that this was for the best but that until now, she had actually been hesitant to recommend I stop. She said I had been like a house of cards when we first met, with alcohol, work, impulsive behaviour and antidepressants all leaning on one another, propping me up. She was reluctant to remove any one of them before I was ready because she feared I might fall in on myself. My foundations were shaky and the life I had built out of a series of dependencies could topple if one were removed too soon. I had to come to terms with myself in order to build a foundation that could withstand the removal of those wobbling interdependencies.

Now that I had begun to do that, and I was growing comfortable in myself, she agreed I was ready to remove the first of my dependencies. I was glad to find that once I took alcohol out of the equation, everything started to grow easier. A few months later, I felt ready to try stopping antidepressants. I will discuss this decision later, but the short answer is that I had been using them for two years and wanted to see, with the oversight of a psychiatrist, how my experiences would feel without them. This is not something I am recommending to anyone else but in my case, medication, like alcohol, was a crutch I used to overcome the anxiety of misunderstanding myself. It was helping me to cope, but I wanted to see if I could process my grief and trauma using what I had learned through therapy and my diagnosis. In a sense, I needed to feel my feelings more fully to understand who I was beneath. While I have never returned to alcohol, I have returned to using antidepressants at certain points since that time. I cannot advise anyone on the use of antidepressant medication, and I hope you understand that my case is not an example but a single, individual experience.

I did find space during that time to come to see aspects of my past in a different light and, in doing so, gained more strength to manage my present. My foundation grew more secure and I could start building new patterns of behaviour on top of it. No more house of cards; I needed structure, but nothing so rigid that it couldn't allow me a little sway. These structures were really just healthy behaviours. You'll see that everything I've introduced into my life as ADHD-friendly practices are ones that most of us can benefit from. They centre on things like sleep, diet and exercise, as well as self-compassion and mindfulness. I believe that if we are going to have norms in our society, these would be the best things to focus on because normalising them would actually benefit us all.

Self-compassion was the starting point for all of my progress, even though in a modern society as ruthlessly comparative and individualistic as ours it can seem non-existent. I had never learned it, practised it or discussed it before that point, but it was only when I learned to speak to myself with love – like the sort of friend that I would be happy to have in my head rather than a critic – that my life improved for the better. To be frank, before I learned to employ self-compassion and to appreciate my difference not as a fault but as individuality, I hated myself and spoke to and about myself accordingly. I just about muddled through life, surviving but never thriving, as my inner critic, the part of me that looked at my thoughts and actions, did not love or care for me.

I only realised with time that if we have one true job on this earth, it is to take care of the person inside of us. The feeling, living being who is much more sensitive, vulnerable and emotional than the external face we present to the world. Once I began to care for my inner self like the continuation of the inner child that it is, the things that previously mattered to me lost meaning and real things grew in their place. We castigate ourselves for not being 'enough', or failing to reach other people's expectations of us, and do not see that we are living a life of punishment on other people's terms, rather than our own. We do not treat ourselves with the empathy that we do the people we love and care for. I would never criticise the people I cared for in the cruel terms I often did myself. How can we be happy, be at peace, without loving ourselves in the way we want others to love us? How can we say we matter if we critique and insult ourselves in a way we wouldn't our worst enemy, let alone our closest, most dependent friend?

I began to care for the person inside of me as if I were a growing, learning child rather than an inadequate man. Whereas all my actions previously had been centred on developing the exterior appearance of a capable adult that satisfied the world, creating turmoil in me, now I had to create an inner life that encouraged peace and steady happy development. I began to put myself to bed at the right time, to eat my greens and to run and play. I want to discuss these things and the approaches I took because I have no doubt that helping our bodies is pivotal if we are to take care of our minds. There are also vital norms to question here. What we have normalised in terms of how we eat, sleep and move is making many of us less happy and less healthy than we would otherwise be, and it would be remiss of me to discuss normality only in terms of thoughts and social ideals without discussing such fundamental things for physical beings.

Sleep was the first aspect of my life that I tried to understand. From what I read, it could play a very significant role in the experience of ADHD, which wasn't a surprise. Sleep is vital to all of us, of course, and anyone who has had to battle through a workday on a bad night's sleep knows how our attention levels and general happiness can be impacted by it. One of the main reasons I would end up with bad sleep was the practice of dopamine-chasing. The human brain and the ADHD brain in particular is wired to crave dopamine hits. This involved pursuing activities that gave me a small hit of satisfaction – anything from a biscuit to an Instagram post. The problem is that most of the activities that provide immediate dopamine hits are at odds with the rest and relaxation that lead to good sleep. If you have ever scrolled through social media before going to bed, you will know how this works.

First, the desire to find the next dopamine-laden post keeps us up. Many tech companies have realised that the best way to keep people on their platform is to provide just the right amount of dopamine at just the right intervals to keep us online. In the same way having a sweet tooth might make someone pursue one extra sweet, our mind makes us pursue another tweet – this keeps us from logging off and bedding down.

Second, many dopamine-chasing behaviours actually energise the brain. In the case of scrolling, the blue light from my phone would trick my mind into feeling like it was time to be awake, but other dopamine-chasing behaviours also act against sleep in other ways. I was eating dopamine-driven foods that contained sugar which kept me awake; the impulsive decision to have one more drink would often make me sleep poorly, and dopamine-heavy TV shows engaged my brain in ways that kept me from feeling restful.

So the very normal desire for dopamine put me at greater risk of sleeping less, and less well when I did, while my ADHD made me extra vulnerable to the impact of poor sleep. I had to completely change my relationship to dopamine-chasing in the hours before I went to bed. I had to normalise a calm, tech-free evening to stop sleeping badly, and only when I could stop sleeping badly could I start sleeping well. It's quite normal to watch telly until the last hour before bed and maybe have a quick scroll on social media before you turn out the light. You might think it strange if you found out a friend gradually turned down the lights in their house as the sun went down, but in the context of our bodies and how they work, that *is* the normal thing to do.

I appreciate that not everything that has worked for me will work for you. I can only describe what has benefitted my life and my mind, and if you leave here with the intention of discovering approaches that work for you, then that is more than enough. The only real takeaway is that it's *normal* to seek dopamine, but we should be conscious of how it impacts important things like how we sleep and eat.

I had to think about my diet a lot as well. The way I eat has been important for managing my sleep and my brain, and everything from what I consume to when I consume it influences how I feel and behave. Like so many aspects of my life, there is a cyclical relationship between my diet and my condition. The nature of my ADHD means I can be impulsive around food and drink. In the past, that meant I would drink far more than I set out to and I would eat for satisfaction as much as nourishment. The short answer is that dopamine-driven eating is generally not good for me. I try to eat to feel good (which is not about dopamine), and I no longer eat to feel *less bad* (which really is). The fact that food is a commodity in a mass market means that our fuel is treated, and marketed, like any other product. And a well-marketed product is one that people want, often, even if it is not good for them.

So in this abnormal world where foods are designed in terms of what they do to our brains rather than how they fuel our bodies, I often found myself seeking comfort foods. These offered guaranteed, quick dopamine hits to counter the anxiety and sadness I felt. They were often sweet, intensive carbohydrates that provided pleasant sensations in the short term but actually made me feel worse in the longer term. Sugar spikes and crashes mirrored not just those highs and lows that I experienced in my attention and mood, but also compounded them. The unfortunate outcome was that I would then be more likely to choose less healthy foods to try to feel better again.

The only way to break the cycle was to reframe my norms around food. Normal food had to be real food: it couldn't have a list of ingredients that looked more like a chemistry project and it basically had to be something that my grandmother would have recognised. It was mostly plants, meat and lots of water. That might sound like an over-simplification but I think the reality goes in the other direction. Food in the twenty-first century is overcomplicated: it's the product of lab testing and research projects, rather than soil and water; it's designed to activate dopamine systems in our minds rather than nourish our bodies.

We have all normalised eating for relief, for convenience and for dopamine, but I think we should try to be conscious of why we need that relief, how inconvenient poor health can be and the role dopamine plays in what we reach for to eat. All our minds can be driven by dopamine and all our bodies can benefit from loosening its grip on our choices.

For a long time, I thought about food and exercise only in terms of my appearance. I wanted to look good. But over time, I realised this was just too simple a way to view such an important aspect of my life. Focusing on appearances was, unsurprisingly, a superficial way of approaching behaviours that impact my whole body and mind, so I tried to think about food in a much more holistic way. Reframing nutrition in terms of what it was doing to my mind really helped, as I am more motivated by managing my condition than I am by 'looking good'. This works for me and, as with so many lifestyle changes, finding one that fits our unique minds, bodies and lifestyles is key.

All of this may lead you to ask where I allow room for some impulsivity in my life. I've told you about my new considered approach to everything from sleep to booze and food, so you may wonder whether I have any space for snap decisions in my new more mindful approach to life. I actually do. I sometimes exercise impulsively. Yes, I know I'm *wild*; I am the party starter and there's no stopping me.

I find exercise to be a fantastic outlet for my natural impulsiveness. If I feel like running, I run. If I feel like going for a stomp, I get outdoors and move with purpose. These are ways of channelling natural impulsivity into behaviours without harmful consequences. Our impulses are not bad in and of themselves, and we should value them and try to own them. But where there is a risk that we are acting *compulsively* or in ways that don't support our happiness or health, it is good to take time to consider our choices. When I have an impulse that I cannot quite place as positive or not, I use my twenty-four-hour rule. This simply means waiting for twenty-four hours after I first had the impulse before I make a decision to act. This gives me enough time to consider whether a decision is the correct one, whether it was a happy, healthy impulse or a compulsion that I would be better off avoiding.

If I can tell immediately that an impulse is a healthy one, however, I'll pursue it gladly. I'll have two smoothies rather than one, I'll paint the town green, call up Toddla T and get him to play a meditation mash-up. I'll exercise impulsively because it makes me less likely to have my impulses manipulated down the line. We're all less likely to compulsively shop, eat or drink if we can create the impulse to exercise instead, because it creates a dopamine hit with a stable run-off. It makes us more likely to sleep and eat better, and it makes me feel good about myself in a way that means I'm less likely to search for self-esteem in self-destructive habits. A lot of people, and ADHDers in particular, turn to cardiovascular exercise as a mental wellbeing tool. I can confidently say it has had a powerful impact on my life and condition. It may be because I have a hunter's body and mind, but in the absence of mammoths I chase PBs. I actually prefer it without the mammoths.

Running gives me a sense of clarity; it is a time when my scattered mind can feel present and the four-second loop is completely engaged in what I am doing. What I experience is sometimes described as a 'flow state'. Now, you could write a whole book on flow states (and Mihaly Csikszentmihalyi did – *Flow: The Psychology of Optimal Experience*), but the short description is that flow states are those where you are so present in a meaningful and enjoyable activity that you become absorbed beyond the point of distraction. You are so present that you are almost absent – or, at least, the part of you that does the thinking and the worrying is. These states are similar to what is described as 'hyperfocus' for ADHDers. It may seem like a contradiction that people who are described as having an 'attention deficit' are associated with extreme focus, but I think that reflects an issue with the naming of ADHD rather than with those of us with it. I can be hyperfocused and give my undivided attention to something over incredibly long timespans. The issue is more that there is a significant disparity between my focus levels when I am engaged versus when I am not. Hyperfocus is the result of deep engagement and a flow state is much the same. Both states can be accessed (for me and many others) through running, but many other physical or mental activities can generate them too.

I do strength training for a complementary, but very different, reason. I find it satisfying because it creates a sense of progress over time, rather than the sense of presence generated through cardio. By taking on an activity like strength training, I can make a positive connection between present action and future progress, which engages my executive function in a healthy way. I described how it can often be difficult to connect up past, present and future in an ordered way, but when you are working with weights there is both a numerical and visual means to track that. Strength training also creates a sense of mind–body connection. By training different parts of my musculature, I become aware of them, their movements and sensations. This does create presence, but more in the sense of location than time. There is not a great deal of research specifically on the subject of how strength training helps the experience of ADHD symptoms, but studies in the general population show that it helps regulate serotonin and dopamine, which are both important chemicals in ADHD minds. This suggests that it is most likely a useful practice and, certainly, in my study of one, it has had consistent positive impacts.

Even before my assessment for ADHD, I did strength-training, but I think the way that its role in my life changed once I was diagnosed is illustrative. Once I understood *why* that training was a positive force in my life, I was able to experience a two-fold benefit, as it is one thing to do something because we like it, but it's more impactful and easier to commit wholeheartedly to it when we understand *why*. In so many aspects of my life, I see how my assessment allowed me to appreciate my positive behaviours and understand my challenging ones. I can enjoy the good impulses with greater depth, and approach my harmful ones with sensitivity, information and forgiveness. I have no reason now to feel inadequate when I struggle but I can access resources when I do.

Even in areas of my life that are not necessarily related to my ADHD, I find that an understanding of it has helped me to become forgiving and to flourish. Maybe being given a reason to pause and reflect on my life has opened up space for me to be kinder to myself. The assessment, diagnosis and results changed my life, but I see now that it was the first time I had really stopped and evaluated my life at all. I had run from myself for so long that I didn't realise I was tired. I had spent so long trying to stretch myself out of the shape I was born into that I didn't realise how much easier being myself could be. When you exist in a society that makes you feel as if your mind is misshapen, you can become so preoccupied fitting its square shape into round holes that you fail to appreciate the shape that you are in. I spent thirty years filing away at the corners of my mind with impulse and alcohol, fight and flight, hard work and hard play, and at no point did I realise that accepting myself might be easier than pretending to be normal.

The first step towards acceptance required me to evaluate both myself and the world with which I felt friction. The next was using the understanding I gained to shape my world into something I could move through smoothly. Now I am taking the step of recounting my history, in an attempt to see it with compassion and to reappraise my experiences with the benefit of knowledge and the security of self-acceptance. It has been a long road that has taken me to this moment, and you will see that there have been a fair number of mishaps and mistakes, but if I have learned anything along the way, it is that no bad can come from greater understanding, even when that feels difficult. I guess you could say that is why I am here.

I have Toddla T to thank for the fork in my road that brought me to the point where I could look back and to forgive. I can credit our chance meeting with my change of path.

Last year a DJ saved my life.

And I'm so glad this is what raving became in my thirties.

2

HOW WERE THINGS
FOR YOU GROWING UP?

Therapy sessions are often built around questions such as the one above. They appear to be simple prompts, invitations to describe a phase or aspect of our lives, but in fact they have a deeper purpose. How we talk about our history, and the process we go through as we evaluate it, often demonstrate a lot about how we think about ourselves. It is by untangling these ways of thinking that we arrive at new perspectives on our past and healthier outlooks on our future.

We're often asked to discuss our childhood in therapy for a number of reasons. The most obvious is that our core beliefs about the world are set in our early years and the behaviours we display in adulthood are responses to how this worldview developed as children. Our ideas of good and bad, what is normal and what is not, are formed early and the ways we modify our behaviour as adults are often the result of how we draw these lines. Some of us can spend a lifetime trying to make our personality fit with the beliefs we formed as children and we struggle as a result. For example, if we are taught as a child that feelings are not to be shared, we can avoid seeking help as an adult. If our childhood experiences showed us that our value as a person is defined by our successes or failures, we may never appreciate our intrinsic value and may hurt ourselves in the pursuit of success to the detriment of our wellbeing. These examples point to the ways in which our childhood nurture and core beliefs can create tensions for us as adults who try to build a life upon them, but also just how damaging it can be for a child to feel ostracised in their early years.

The messages that children hear about themselves at this very early stage are also hugely influential. It is estimated that by the age of five, a child with ADHD has received around 20,000 negative comments as a result of their neurodiversity. This could contribute to the rejection sensitivity and dysphoria (a state of unease within ourselves) that many ADHD people experience and is often described as one of the most challenging aspects of our experience. There is a truly wonderful initiative run by the Princess of Wales through her Early Childhood campaign that really engages with the issue of early years development and the stigmatisation of children at a time when their neuroplasticity (the ability of the brain to change itself) is greatest. Our sense of value, of being loved or appreciated in those first five years can mean the difference between seeing the world as a threatening or welcoming place, and ourselves as intrinsically valuable or defective. I am not an expert in childrearing or child psychology, so I am reticent to discuss specific norms in those fields, but I would say that this shows how deeply important it is that we as a society consider how we approach very young children and their development.

These are questions of nurture but I also find discussions of childhood interesting because they open up space to talk about our nature. This is a subject fraught with debate and there is really no definitive answer on how the sliding scale between the two should be calibrated, but, while I am not concerned with academic questions about nature and nurture, I am interested in how appreciating both can help us to become more accepting of ourselves and more forgiving. Aspects of our mind and behaviour that we mistakenly describe as defects or limitations can often be much better understood as features of our character. While we need not see ourselves as 'broken' or 'fixed', or excuse bad behaviour as a result of our nature, we can certainly free ourselves from unnecessary pain when we accept certain parts of ourselves rather than struggle with how we believe we *should* be.

There are many aspects of my behaviour in childhood that reflect the person that I became. Aristotle supposedly said, 'Give me the child until he is seven, and I will show you the man', and it is my hope that showing you the child I was at seven might help us both understand the man I am today. I was sensitive and energetic. I was deeply motivated when my attention was captured and miles away when it was not. I liked fast things and long summer days. Show that child to Aristotle and he would have no problem picking my adult self out of a line-up.

I was born in West Wales, where my parents had bought a smallholding because they wanted to raise my two brothers and me in the countryside. This was a thoughtful decision on their part. They could have moved somewhere smaller in the town and probably made their lives easier financially and practically, but they stretched themselves and took on a larger mortgage so that we would all have space to roam. Instead of holidays or meals out, we had fields to run in. Their money went towards paying off their bills and creating a pleasant space for their growing boys, so we spent our weekends and holidays together on the land, with the odd trip to the beach when the sun reared its head and shone upon the Welsh coast.

It was a traditional rural setting in more ways than one. Our area had a lot of Welsh-speakers and I attended bilingual primary and secondary schools. We don't often consider the depth and variety of language and culture on the British Isles, but our area was steeped in it. The saints and mythological figures were as much a feature of the landscape as the rocky cliffs and sandy bays of Pembrokeshire or the rolling fields of Carmarthenshire. Those places and those stories are forever a part of me, even though I have lost a lot of my Welsh in the fifteen years since I finished studying and living amid the language. I intend to improve my Welsh again, as there's something very powerful about the ties to our history and community that a language creates.

Speaking Welsh was certainly discouraged in my parents' generation, so they never learned it, but they took pride in our history and the fact that their children spoke it in Carmarthenshire. Our house had a Welsh name, Panteg, while the garden out front was called The Clunk, which is nonsense. A few years ago, I asked my mother how it got that name and discovered it was a word I had made up as a small child who found it easier and more satisfying to say than 'garden'.

The Clunk and Panteg were a huge part of my world as a child; in fact, they felt like the whole world to me. Beyond that little world of mine, which seemed so big to me as a small person, there was the local village of Capel Dewi, which seemed large but to a cosmopolitan eye would appear anything but. It contained, and still contains, a village hall, tennis court and forty or so houses. No post office, no pub. The community is close knit and kind, with agriculture and mutual support tying the people together. The next village along was Nantgaredig, where my primary school was. This was slightly larger, with two pubs and a post office.

The world grew as you travelled outward from my home, with the family-sized Panteg growing into the small community of Capel Dewi, on towards the town of Carmarthen and next, the world. Carmarthen town has a claim to being the oldest in Wales, with evidence of Roman amphitheatres dotted around the banks of the River Tywi and a proud history as Wales's major urban centre in the sixteenth and seventeenth centuries. It's nothing like that now, but it was a great place to go and meet friends once I was old enough to make the twenty-minute drive myself as a teenager.

These were the places that formed me and though I now live on the banks of the Thames rather than the Tywi, much of it remains within me. These were the places where my nurture took place and my nature took form. I was the first child of Anthony and Jane, a police officer and bank manager. My father joined the police in his late twenties after spending his teens and young adulthood working on go-karts and cars with his own father. Blood is thicker than water, but not as thick as petrol (chemists, let me know!), and in my family the love of speed goes back generations. I can trace that line at least as far back as my grandfather (although those Roman amphitheatres may have contained a George grinning on a chariot for all I know). He raced go-karts at national and international levels and, as anyone who has followed the careers of Formula 1 professionals knows, those small vehicles are a big deal, providing the gateway to elite motorsport worldwide.

I share my grandfather's comfort at high speeds. As a child, I would ride scrambler bikes around the fields or take a three-wheeler Honda trike over bumps and into ditches without a care in the world. I have always been drawn to the adrenaline and the (seemingly contradictory) calm of moving at high speeds. Then, as now, moving fast makes my mind feel slower and more present. Motorsport professionals and hobbying speed enthusiasts I have spoken to often say the same thing. They are at rest when they travel at the edge of what is possible. Peter Hickman, who holds records at the Isle of Man TT, said on the Stompcast that he is most calm on the limit. Peaceful, even.

This might be a feature of my ADHD or it might simply be that different minds and bodies find joy in different places and at different speeds. When you are strapped into a brain that moves faster than is comfortable though, an even faster vehicle can help it find its place. I've ridden at up to 180mph on a track, and I can honestly say that time and space moved slower and more predictably for me at that speed than it does at the pace of daily life. When your mind lacks brakes, you are grateful for a throttle. (At least, I am.)

From what I'm told, this state of mind, this 'lack of brakes', was present from very early in my life. I was an anxious baby, prone to crying and in need of a lot of attention and comfort. I can only imagine my newborn dependence and lack of mobility was a frustration, and I cried out for the freedom of movement upon which my mind still so relies. Once I was able to walk and talk, I did so quickly and without much regard for my, or anyone else's, safety, walking for the first time at nine months by holding onto our dog's fur for balance! My mother tells me she would often find I had climbed on top of the washing machine when I was hardly able to walk to it. When I was three years old, she had to pacify a passing builder who was shocked to find a very small child up in a tree in front of the house.

My father, like my grandfather, shares my love of speed and high-pressure situations, and I think our decisions to both become emergency responders ties into that somehow. As a police officer or an accident and emergency doctor, you take part in the professional and social equivalent of racing at high speed. Events and accidents come at you like corners, and you apply brakes only when necessary because speed of thought and action are of the essence. He is fantastic under pressure and I'm glad he found a career that so matched his skills. I think he too is on the ADHD spectrum, as the joys and challenges he experiences are very similar to mine, but I am still trying to get him to do an assessment. As a man of his time and stoic to a fault, he is difficult to convince but he's only sixty-seven so we still have time.

Mental health and neurodivergence were not often discussed by my parents' generation, and this was mostly still the case in West Wales when I was growing up. I think my mother and father both experienced anxiety (as many of us do) but had very different ways of dealing with it. My father is one to keep a lid on his emotions – to a man born in the fifties in rural Wales, that is perfectly normal to him and right, even if it causes him discomfort. The norms of a father, of a rural man in Wales and a police officer, all combined to dictate that he should always present a strong and stable face to the world, but I am in no doubt that created a certain internal pressure.

These norms are being challenged today. Police officers are being given more room to recognise the stress and psychological strain that they face as a consequence of doing their jobs and more measures are being put in place to offer counselling and outlets for them to discuss their experiences. Men more broadly are realising that the norms of 'strength as silence' and 'masculinity as inscrutability' have had their time. I can feel the change. Men's mental health is a subject close to my heart and it fills me with hope that a generation growing up in West Wales now has a better understanding of it than mine ever did. There are still many for whom the approaches of my father's generation would seem normal, in the sense of being right, so there's still work to be done by those of us who disagree.

My mother experienced her anxiety differently. Rather than seeking the supposedly masculine form of self-control my father practised, she leaned into the image of a maternal family fixer that women were often led to believe was their role. As a mother and a woman, you *had* to be OK and you had to make sure everyone else was too, because problems were there to be sorted and situations to be controlled. You kept the peace. This still contains an element of repression. If we are trying to solve everyone else's problems, we rarely have time to acknowledge our own, and we tend to focus on symptoms rather than causes. I sympathise with my mum: she bore a great weight of responsibility and her parenting approach was the norm in her world and her time, but I'm pleased to see things changing both for parents and their children. I'm glad there's an improved understanding that taking care of others at the expense of taking care of ourselves is misguided, because we can only care well when we are well. That the peace is not worth keeping if turmoil is driven inward.

My parents created a beautiful home and a caring environment for smart and sensitive children, but it was often difficult for me to fit into the routine and order of a traditional family. I think this is quite a common experience for children with ADHD. I struggled to keep to the rules and meet the standards that my parents expected of me, and sometimes this could cause friction. They were faced with a child who didn't seem to be committed to doing things the correct way, and I was faced with a world that didn't yet appreciate that ADHD is not a lack of commitment but a neurodevelopmental condition. My parents were loving, thoughtful and understanding, but without awareness of, or access to, information about my condition and the sensitivity that came with it, there were always going to be aspects of my behaviour that they struggled with.

I worried a lot as a child and I turned to self-soothing as a response. There was a prominent school of thought in child psychology and parenting in the first half of the twentieth century that this was a healthy thing for a child to do. The American psychologist John B. Watson, the 'father of behaviourism', normalised a view that an over-reliance on parental nurture and communication was bad for childhood development. My parents didn't necessarily subscribe to Watson's view but I wonder whether I internalised some of society's acceptance of Watson's thinking as a child. I didn't open up or share about my anxiety, or communicate about the prevailing sense of my own difference, because I grew up in a culture that didn't expect children to do that. Instead, I kept my discomfort inside and tried to calm my overactive mind. When I was anxious or needed to sleep, I would blast the hairdryer on full volume as a sort of white noise to override the static in my mind. It was escapism and it felt necessary to me, but it was not a solution.

We now know that love, affection and healthy communication are vital for a child's development. The solution is to normalise the discussion of discomfort and anxiety for children, which is something I am committed to. Like adults, children will seek to suppress their anxiety as long as stigma exists, and as long as they lack approaches to understand and explain it. If we do not have the language and permission to describe difficult mental health, both adults and children will try to soothe themselves in whatever way they can, when it would be far more impactful to learn to understand ourselves and soothe one another.

The hairdryer was one of many ways that I sought solace as a child who felt at odds with the world but, like most of my approaches, it centred on shutting it out, so I often sought the safety of being alone in my room. While the hairdryer treatment relied on a manageable form of stimulation to override the chaos of an over-stimulating world, the quiet and control of my own room was all about the absence of it. I struggled with the complexity of the world outside those four walls because social life and its expectations came into conflict with my own ability to process them. It always followed the same pattern: I would become over-stimulated and retreat into myself, which would cause people to become frustrated with me, in turn making me even more anxious. I knew that people were taking issue with my behaviour but I lacked the language to explain why. In the space left by this explanatory gap, I would fill myself up with anxious questions. *Do people like me? What do they really think of me? Am I enough?*

I look back and feel sadness and sympathy for that small boy. Contemporary norms around communicating with children, neurodivergence and mental health would suggest this was not a question of being liked but an issue of not being understood. My difference did not equate to my value because we all have intrinsic worth regardless of our relationship to the norms that surround us. I was a neurodivergent child growing up in social and educational circumstances that couldn't recognise or support me. I was applying the logic of personal value to explain the friction I felt with a world I couldn't understand, and I continued to do so in the space left by a culture that didn't think it normal to take time to understand children's thoughts.

The other great question that circled my small mind in the safety of my room was, 'Do I fit in?' *This* was closer to the point. At least the question of fitting in makes room for the reality that there is something to fit into and it could open up to the realisation that society is often at fault if a child feels that they do not belong. Still, I was a long way from reaching the view I have now, which is that the world treats certain ways of being as normal but that difference doesn't mean you lack value or don't fit. Moreover, it should not be normal for a child to decide such things and not have the opportunities to discuss them with trusted adults at home, school or in the community. I was not ready to diagnose problems with the world and instead saw myself as the problem.

Neurodivergence and social anxiety are a troublesome combination. The structure of your mind both makes you different and terribly afraid of being different. Without the language of neurodivergence, you don't really have a way to untangle the knot, but I think that as a society, we are growing in our understanding. Recognition and identification can often seem like small progress in the absence of true support, and, while this is true, the simple fact of being aware of difference existing – that it isn't just you who feels like you don't fit in – can have a transformative effect. I think it would have for me.

I am proud to have been a confused and socially anxious child who became a public figure who tries to speak about mental health. The ways in which I am different have provided me with a platform to advocate for new norms, approaches and ways of thinking. I am familiar with the isolation that a lack of public health provisions can entail for people who don't fit into the 'normal' categories as well as experience of treating people who have fallen through the net, so I hope that gives me a degree of perspective and empathy.

The fact that as a socially anxious person, I have chosen to speak out so publicly may seem strange. I'm not recognised enough for it to be a constant occurrence but there is no denying that I get attention in public places that I wouldn't have received before I appeared on television and I do find that challenging. In fact, I think a lifetime of social anxiety has prepared me quite well for the feeling of being stared at! I spent so long thinking 'I don't fit in' and coming to terms with it, that standing out, is something I have practised.

It also helps that some of the self-soothing approaches I adopted as a child and teenager continue to offer me solace as an adult. I am not talking about the hairdryer (which I do sometimes still use), but things like spending time with animals and in nature. These have been my mental health practices since long before I knew what mental health was. I turned to my dogs for companionship and comfort as a child, and to this day, my dog, Rolo, offers me the same sense of soothing. Animals can be a source of calm and joy to human minds of many different shapes, from socially anxious and neurodiverse children to the emotionally bottled-up fathers who start out saying they don't want a pet but end up loving and nurturing their pet with a freedom they may never have enjoyed with other humans.

Pets have also been shown to provide great social and psychological solace to people in a variety of therapeutic situations. There are dogs that support people through grief, post-traumatic stress disorders and Alzheimer's, while children on the autism spectrum often benefit from the companionship of pets and the positive social experiences they can provide. All of these varied minds benefit from the supportive, uncritical company of animals and, even better, they help us get outside.

I think this is first (and forgive me if these things seem obvious) because dogs are sociable but uncritical. With a pet like Rolo, there is no reason to worry about whether you are behaving in line with social norms, because in a dog's eyes, their humans fit in just fine, particularly if they have food and sticks, which I find to be a manageable set of expectations.

Second, dogs are great because they have a very broad energy spectrum. Dogs can achieve great excitement and activity as well as an almost preternatural state of calm. Their animalistic appreciation of running, jumping and playing is something that modern society mostly discourages in adults, while their ability to truly relax is something many of us can only dream of in the hectic, attention-grabbing world we live in. Dogs experience highs and lows of energy and activity that I genuinely find inspiring, and a great antidote to a culture that keeps us in a constant state of low-level stimulation and vigilance.

It may sound odd to have aspirations to be more like a dog, but hey, I have no fears about being odd at this point. In fact, I've heard a lot of people extolling the virtue of 'being more dog'. Whether it is in how we exercise, shrug off disappointment or focus on being in the moment, to be 'more dog' is not the worst piece of advice you could receive. So run when you feel like it, respond to life's treats rather than disappointments and exist in the moment. It's your dog-given right.

The natural world *was* my world growing up and, just as my room could provide a safe space, so did the fields and forests around me. Nature was and will always be fundamentally calming – in a social world that is unpredictable and moves at an overwhelming pace, the passage of time in the natural world is the complete opposite. Nature can move at a pace of seconds or millions of years, depending on which time frame you decide to tap into. It can be engrossing in its minutiae or awe-inspiring in its grandeur. It can be a gateway to meditation or to seeing the sciences in action. It simply *is*, and that means you can draw from it the form of stimulation you need. Whether you want to study mountains or molehills, the sort of mind that sometimes makes one out of the other can find in it a scale and pace that creates a sense of comfort.

The natural world provided the backdrop to most of my happiest memories of childhood. The feeling of waking up on a summer's day and seeing the sun – always a sign of a good day ahead. Climbing trees and hay bales, riding scramblers around in the mud or running over sand dunes to the sea. Being outside, with space to move among landscapes that are both peaceful and energising, created in me a sense of belonging where I too could be as peaceful or as energetic as I needed to be.

It also made me feel capable, which was not something I often experienced at that age. There was movement involved but it was not sport, where I lacked the confidence to put myself forward for team games. There was so much to pay attention to but no educational framework to make my attention span feel like a problem. There was stimulation but no judgement. In nature, my social anxiety was not a factor as it was in sport and school. I discovered later that both of those things could be sources of great joy and meaning for me, but in my early years, they were too fraught with complexity. It is a shame that I took so long to discover that they could be good for me and that I could draw a sense of accomplishment from them.

In part, I struggled with team sports as a child because of my social anxiety; I felt uncertain at the lack of control they entailed but I also simply found new experiences difficult in general. To this day, transitions are not a strong point for me. At various junctures in my life, I have considered quitting some new pursuit simply because the transitional period has been overwhelming. I found the move from primary to secondary school difficult, moving to London to become a doctor was a hard time and even changing roles as a trainee was enough to make me doubt my ability to adapt. This is a fact of my personality that I have learned to account for and mediate. I have to retain certain comforts and routines, and I have to give myself some breathing space while I adjust to a new set of circumstances, be that a holiday or a big professional challenge.

I understand now that this means retaining a healthy base. Which I achieve through a routine of sleep, exercise and nutrition, allied to a consciousness that in any transition, the difficult time will pass. The nature of my mind is such that I can catastrophise a difficult moment into an apparently terminal situation. So I must remind myself that the moment I am in is not permanent, that the difficulties presented by the change will pass, and only then am I able to see it for what it is and move towards comfort. Soon, what is difficult and new will become routine and my experience of it will be as straightforward as what I had grown accustomed to previously.

I may be a creature of habit, but life requires us to progress and learn that new experiences can become habits in time. This was the case at school, in work and in my daily behaviours. While I could genuinely follow the same routine every day, my longer-term goals constantly require me to confront new experiences. If I only ever aimed to be the guy who went to the same coffee shop, gym and workplace every day, I could live within the same regimented routine, but my aspirations won't allow it, so I have to be flexible. I need routine but I crave freedom too.

My brother, Elliott, recently spoke to me about a difficulty he was having with a transition. He was in the RAF and when he left, he was given a dream job opportunity in Germany. After a few weeks, he was already finding the reality to be different from the expectations he'd had and was considering coming home. It became clear to us both as we discussed it that it was not that the situation was a problem, but the transition. In fact, when we are struggling with the supposed reality of a new situation, we are not confronting the reality of it at all because our first impressions are usually very different from what it will actually turn out to be like. How we feel about a place *at first* is never quite the same as how we feel about it after we have grown comfortable within it. We agreed on that and he stayed, eventually growing to enjoy the experience.

He is similar to me in his relationship to change but in most other ways we are very different. We were born four years apart and even though our circumstances were incredibly similar, our characters are not. Whereas I struggled to be accepted by the education system, he rebelled against it. We had similar challenges with organisation and attention, but he decided to see the school system as the problem, rather than himself, and so he built a life in which he didn't have to struggle with academia as I did. We were not particularly close as children but we are closer now because we accept and understand each other's differences.

My youngest brother, Llŷr, was born six years after Elliott and ten years after me. I helped to choose his name, which is Welsh for the god of the sea. Llŷr was a wonderful boy, the spitting image of me, with a similar sensitivity. He was much younger than Elliott and me, so our relationship was different from that of us two older brothers. When we were riding motorbikes, he was toddling along after us, and by the time I was leaving for university, he was still only eight.

I think that we would all have benefitted from conversations about how we approached change, control and social anxiety as children. This would have improved our experience of childhood but also provided us with tools that we could use throughout our lifetimes. I now dedicate a great deal of my time to opening up avenues for children to discuss their mental wellbeing, and to access approaches for managing and improving it. We have moved past the mute acceptance of mental health challenges and the self-destructive stoicism of silence, but now we have a duty to equip people with the tools to address the challenges they face and feel better. This should begin early, and it should take place at home and at school. The norm that children should be seen and not heard should finally be left behind.

I certainly believe I would have gained a lot from more open conversations about mental health as a child. While self-soothing can be helpful, it shouldn't be the only option, and communication about anxiety is often a key step in developing the resources to process it. Discussions of mental wellbeing have a positive role in any relationship and I don't think our interactions with children should be any different. My experiences of anxiety and neurodivergence as a child were compounded by the sense that these things made me abnormal, and while anxiety and neurodivergence are complex states of mind, notions of normality are not. By discussing a child's feelings, we can better understand their fear of difference and provide reassurance, before approaching the provisions that we must offer to respond to anxiety or neurodivergence. We must not allow the fear of difference to compound them.

I think that there's room for more discussion of what a 'normal' childhood actually looks like. The historical norm was that children had a lot of freedom and were largely left to their own devices, but received strict punishments and very little explanation of why. They were not raised to think about their mental wellbeing but they did engage in a lot of behaviours that we now understand contribute to good mental wellbeing, like exercise, a sense of agency and community. Now we have children who are taught about mental health but live in a way that is often not conducive to it. The opportunities for exploration, freedom and exercise are more limited than ever. Which means we have normalised openness about mental wellbeing but closed the door on many things which support it. In today's terms, my childhood was not normal. I had a healthier environment in terms of the freedom to take risks but a much less healthy one in terms of my ability to speak about how I was feeling. I am proud of the progress that has been made on one of these norms but I think we need to be conscious that on others, we have travelled backwards.

If we can raise children in a way that allows them to understand and speak about their mental wellbeing and *also* experience the freedom to do the things that support it, we could combine the best of the old and new ways. This will take a concerted effort: children should have safe spaces to explore and parents should feel reassured that their children are stepping out into a world that is not a threat to them. In cities, this means maintaining our community spaces like parks, ensuring our roads are safe and re-establishing a sense of community whereby we all realise that we have responsibility for children who enter public spaces without their parents. In rural areas, we should protect those green spaces, waterways and common areas like sports pitches where children can go to explore and have fun.

I can only imagine how our society could be transformed by raising children with a healthy degree of freedom, a good grounding in mental health and wellbeing, and tools for processing the stresses associated with it. Our communities, workplaces and healthcare systems would change as the adults of tomorrow entered them with greater understanding and self-compassion. By improving the experiences of children today, we can raise happier, healthier adults tomorrow.

So we must think like Aristotle and provide the child of seven with the resources they will need as an adult. Because what is the future but what we decide to teach the children of today?

3

DID YOU ENJOY SCHOOL?

I often felt like a problem at school and for a long time, school felt like a problem to me. I wasn't wrong. Through school, I was being introduced to a society's ways of working, its expectations around order, attention and focus. As it became clear to me that my ways of thinking didn't match up to these, I saw school as evidence that I might never really fit in. For the majority of my education experience (up to age sixteen), my schools valued obedience, repetition and organisation, which are all valuable traits that don't come easily to me. As a result, I assumed that I was simply not very good at school and would most likely struggle in the years afterwards. From sixteen onwards, though, I was exposed to different education priorities – those of insight, autonomy and creativity. As it turned out, I was quite good at these aspects. When the education system broadened its image of what a capable student could be, I broadened my horizons.

How we experience school is important because our education system is a microcosm of our society. If we accept the idea that the beliefs and skills of our future leaders are determined by the education they receive as children, then we can reasonably say that it is the start of future societies too. How we design our schools tells us what we value in our culture. If we seek happy, healthy, self-sufficient adults, our education system will need to teach children about wellbeing and health through self-directed learning over rote memorisation. If our society prioritises order, then rigour, hierarchy and conformity will be valued over autonomy or wellbeing.

The significance of resources in this conversation is not lost on me. Whichever route we go down, our political system has to fund education providers adequately to carry out their plans. While my primary school was good, my secondary school was poorly resourced and under-performing, and I often see through my work with education charities how financial constraints are the greatest impediment to providing children with the support they need. No amount of charitable endeavour or education philosophy can overcome an absence of political will and resources. The most progressive education system cannot grow organically out of one that is under-resourced, and nor can it be shaped from one that prioritises results over wellbeing. If test scores and attainment targets are the measure by which schools are judged, rather than their ability to raise mentally fit, resilient children, wellbeing will often be compromised at the expense of performance. Teachers too will suffer.

To illustrate, let's take the example of the two education systems I described above, which could loosely be described as 'progressive' and 'traditional'. The traditional model is the one we all know: one size fits all, rote learning for examinations in a time- and resource-poor environment. The progressive model encourages self-directed learning, with examinations as a tool to understand progress rather than the goal; differentiation for students who learn and think differently; and an emphasis on mental and physical wellbeing as the primary goal of education. Which do we think is preferable?

For me it is the so-called progressive model, and I will use my experiences of education to explain why. My experience is of course of the former. But if we are to look at this only in the context of providing affordable public services, which of the two do we think is more cost effective? Most people assume it is the traditional model: strict, structured environments with a high student to teacher ratio that keeps staff costs down and simplifies the delivery of education through a sink-or-swim approach to children: you either fit with the process or fail, and this is cheaper than keeping everyone afloat. I am not sure this is true and would in fact argue that a system that fails teachers and children is the most expensive there could be. If we burn out our teachers, then the education sector's savings are simply the healthcare system's losses (in 2024, 87 per cent of teachers lost sleep over stress and 76 per cent pointed to the school inspections' programme run by Ofsted – the Office for Standards in Education, Children's Services and Skills – as having a negative impact on their wellbeing and mental health).

Our education system is not simply a microcosm of our society, it is a whole generation's first point of contact with it, so any cost savings we try to make can really never be understood without considering the costs to society at large. Keeping children in classrooms all the time will save money, but it will also impact their physical health – children are happier and healthier when given more time to run around outside. If they are never taught to understand their mental and emotional health, they are much more likely to develop struggles with mental illness throughout their lives, without the tools to get better. There is a better way: educate and empower children and young adults with the skills they need to build mental fitness, and the emotional literacy to understand and name what they are experiencing when struggles first appear. Happy children are much more likely to be able to engage in learning and contribute to the school environment.

I think the decision to follow 'traditional' educational approaches is as much about historic norms as it is about funding. It is much harder to change something than continue as we are, even if it means making the same mistakes. Our vision of a classroom, of thirty or forty students to one teacher, of strict curricula and tiny people in suits, goes back to the Victorian era. It is no coincidence that this was the last time there was a genuine significant shift in education provision, and I believe that we find it hard to imagine a school in any other way. It's only by envisioning an alternative to what we consider normal, however, that we can see the limitations of what we have.

Why would we persevere with our current approach if it is neither healthier nor cheaper? It could only be because it appears *simpler*. The authoritarian education idea is an economy of scale, the only feasible approach to keeping thirty children in line with only one or two supervising adults, when both time and space are constrained. It would take a lot of work to create classrooms that are physically and mentally healthy places in which children and teachers can thrive, but the most impactful change would come from having more staff.

Wouldn't it make sense to have *a lot* more grown-ups in each classroom? Enough staff to ensure that teachers had the time, space and discretion to support children and themselves properly. The most significant breakthroughs I made in my education came when there was a supportive adult taking time to explain why I wasn't making the progress I should be. I was a child who learned and worked in a different way to others, and I assumed that this was because there was something wrong with me when what I needed was a responsible adult to look at my situation and explain how I could make my mind work towards my goals. This takes time and money, and it takes staff. The only way an education system can support a diverse range of learning styles and minds is by having enough staff to offer individual support. I was an outlier and stretched public services do not have the resources to focus on outliers. Normality is, in many senses, a resource issue but when this issue is in education, it has the potential to alienate and problematise whole generations of children, with worrying consequences for their futures as individuals and for our future as a society.

Many of the challenges I see teachers and students face can be brought back to the idea of norms and of standardisation. We lack the resources to offer education that accounts for diverse minds and learning styles, but we are also drawn to standardised curricula and regular examinations because they provide us with a simple, *generalisable* approach to understanding young people's progress.

We evaluate children regularly against a norm of progress and we rate schools based on the norms that have been established by bodies like Ofsted. In many areas, these approaches are now being questioned. While many people believed that more regular examinations of pupils and evaluations of schools would provide more feedback and insight, it has instead created more conservative learning environments. When we fear getting things wrong, we are less likely to attempt innovative approaches that might get things right. Strict academic standards mean we fail to teach skills such as teamwork, self-directed learning and inquisitiveness. We try to make all students exam-ready, and this can limit the ways in which we teach life skills that are integral to becoming a well-rounded person but hard to examine through a GCSE.

I struggled at school from quite early on because my style of learning failed to fit with a norm that prioritises obedience over inquisitiveness and passivity over activity. When something interested me, I would focus well and complete tasks quickly, but if I struggled to understand a key component or became disengaged, I would soon grow distracted. The expectation that we would sit quietly for long periods of time and retain focus without regular interaction and stimulation was very difficult for me. While I could be quite engaged in class and enjoyed answering questions and contributing to discussions, I seriously struggled with writing. My handwriting was (and is) terrible because I lacked the focus to gather my thoughts and write methodically. We sometimes forget that writing is a craft that children have to work hard to develop – a mixture of fine motor skills and joined-up thinking that requires a great deal of attention. This is where I fell down; my lack of focus and concentration made me prone to errors and I could sense that the adults around me thought I had a problem.

ADHD was never considered as an explanation for my learning challenges in childhood. There was a lack of cultural awareness around neurodivergence but also little time available to get to the root of my difficulties. I was simply thought of as a child who struggled with presentation, concentration and attention. I was 'easily distracted' or 'unfocused', always one euphemism away from being understood. The truth was that I was so lost in anxious thoughts and imaginary problems that I was creating very real ones for myself.

My inattention often frustrated teachers. My earliest memory of this happening occurred St Dwynwen's day. St Dwynwen is the Welsh saint of love. I much prefer her to Cupid, as her intentions seem less manipulative and far more human. She was so unlucky in love that she gave up and became a nun, spending her life praying for true lovers to have better luck than she did. Her noble and selfless approach makes Cupid look rather childish and has the added benefit of requiring neither bows nor arrows. I remember I zoned out as our lesson progressed before refocusing for long enough to put my hand up and ask whether she was a boy or a girl. It seemed a reasonable question to me but frustrated my teacher, who thought I was being deliberately difficult, making a mockery of his attempt to teach us about the saint. He was clearly annoyed, in the way that caregivers often are at children with ADHD. They can naturally feel ignored or underappreciated, forgetting (or not realising) that their frustration is the result of another person's disability. This in turn can lead to people with ADHD and ASD (autism spectrum disorder) being heavily criticised, affecting their confidence. In the example above, I was singled out, which left me feeling stupid, ashamed and unlikely to ask questions in class in future.

The more experiences like this I had as a child, the more I would try to stay under the radar. My mixture of inquisitiveness and distractibility had never seemed to be a problem until primary school. So I learned what some people would call tact but others in the neurodivergent community call 'masking'. This is the practice of hiding aspects of your neurodivergence in the hope of making your life easier.

I think that many people mask to an extent, whether they are neurodivergent or not. We may have a professional mask, which is a version of ourselves that we can put on at work to hide our fears and doubts. Many men I have known rely on a mask of masculinity to avoid presenting their vulnerability to the world. It is a costume of competence, consistency and strength that comes at the expense of authenticity and keeps us from engaging with and supporting one another. Our masks are simply devices that we all wear to meet the standards of normality that we believe society has set for us. We think that because we wear similar masks, we are all similar, when in reality we are all similar because we believe we need to wear them. If we could remove our masks we could see our shared vulnerability and collective abnormality.

My ADHD masking at school was clearly unsuccessful as I was moved into a special educational needs group from the age of eight or nine. In a sense, this was correct: my educational needs did require some special consideration but unfortunately all this designation entailed was lower expectations. I was given less to learn rather than different – and more suitable – approaches to learning.

This is an example of the unfortunate bind that low staff-to-student ratios and limited classroom support leaves teachers and pupils in. The nature of my challenges and solutions to them could only have become clear with staff who were trained to see the signs of neurodivergence, who could educate me on how to flourish as a neurodivergent person, and joined-up thinking to address how our school system prioritises a one-dimensional learning approach. I can only imagine how these early interventions would have transformed my life and the challenges I could have later avoided.

I did flourish eventually but my experiences got worse before they got better. The early years of secondary school can be hard for any child, but for pupils like me they can be particularly difficult. By the time I was in year 7 I had learned to hide myself and avoid provoking the ire of my teachers, but I had started having problems with other students. My secondary school was tough, a coeducational facility that catered to students from the town and country in Carmarthenshire, and struggled to keep a lid on tensions and manage problematic behaviour. There were a lot of fights and a lot of bullying. I think I was picked on for being sensitive, for being odd, for being me, but it is hard to understand a perpetrator's logic when you are a victim. I still marvel at the accuracy with which teenagers diagnose any oddness or outgroup behaviour in their peers. My bullies lasered in on me from day one and designated me a nerd. I felt short-changed though, as this nerd was rarely even appreciated by teachers.

I have no doubt now that the children who were making my life difficult were probably processing or unloading some difficulties of their own. A lot of them came from challenging home environments and very few children set out to be cruel for cruelty's sake. This is another case where schools need resources such as dedicated healthcare professionals, because as it stands, teachers are simply too busy meeting the demands of examinations and curricula to address bullying adequately. My work with The Diana Foundation has made me aware of the prevalence of bullying in schools. A third of children experience it, with those figures higher for children on free school meals or with a disability. We need to admit that, unfortunately, it is 'normal' to be bullied and recognise that we normalise bullying behaviours in many parts of adult society (think about reality television, social media, tabloid journalism and you'll see what I mean).

Conflict resolution is only one aspect of fixing the problem, as the root causes of bullying can only be addressed if we consider the unhappiness that leads to bullying as well as that which results from it. So I believe that we should prioritise counselling for both the victims and perpetrators of bullying. School counsellors and therapists are essential to this. If you have doubts about how we can fund such staff, I want to remind you that we fund teenage mental health care but only when it becomes problematic enough to engage the social and emergency services. It would be cheaper and more effective to provide support earlier, and the earliest and most effective point at which we can intervene in a child's life is in school.

Arguably, the greatest intervention in my school life came from a teacher who believed in me. His name was Mr Harris and around year ten, he began to take a keen interest in my progress. Mr Harris seemed to believe that beneath my dysfunctional and disordered relationship with the school system, there was a capable young man waiting to be engaged – and he told me as much. He was a senior teacher who had no issue managing student behaviour because we were passionately engaged, giving him the freedom to allow for more discussion in his lessons. He created a fast-paced intellectual atmosphere and because he was safe in the knowledge that order would be maintained, he could allow for a certain amount of healthy disorder that was not normal in my experience. We debated questions of ethics and moral philosophy and I started to come alive. I realised that sitting still (intellectually) was not always a prerequisite for intelligence, and that I could be sharp and insightful when stimulated. I realised that my learning style was legitimate and had only felt abnormal because no one had yet had the time to engage it. I left every lesson motivated and emboldened by learning and when Mr Harris saw that, he harnessed it to make me believe in myself. That is a testament to his ability but also to the impact a teacher can make when they aren't weighed down by the pressure of their position. Mr Harris passed away recently but I know that in my life, and the lives of others who he believed in when we were children, his profound impact lives on.

The acronym VARK is often used to describe the four types of learner: *visual* (seeing), *auditory* (listening and speaking), *reading* (and writing) and *kinesthetic*. Most of my schooling fell into the

listening part of auditory learning and the reading or writing styles.
I think this has been normalised as the go-to learning approach
in British schools due to the resource and time constraints we
previously discussed. It is hard to have a learning environment
that prioritises speaking unless we have small group sizes, where
discussions can be manageable and orderly. Kinesthetic learners
need space, physical representations of the learning materials and a
teacher who has the time and ability to communicate concepts with
movement, which is realistically rarely possible in our education
system as it is. Mr Harris was a passionate teacher for whom class
control wasn't a challenge and, as a result, he could prioritise
speaking and a degree of kinesthetic learning. This was not normal
but it really made me feel normal, as learning became far more
accessible.

It was around that time, and with the benefit of that new self-
esteem, that another important step in my school career took place.
I made a proper friend. Up until that point I had a few mates but not
the sort of era-defining teenage friendship that I found with Adam,
the sort that can change your whole perspective on life. When I tell
you I made a friend, that might sound like small progress but what
if I told you that I made a *really cool* friend, a rugby-playing friend, a
'girls want to date him' sort of friend. Now do you see what this could
mean to the perennial outcast of the lower-school corridors? It was
the stuff of teenage movies. The coolest guy in the year decided that
I might just be cool too. Of course, it kind of makes me cringe when
I think about it, but whatever!

It genuinely changed my life. What started with some self-belief imparted by a brilliant teacher sparked the light of a friendship, and I started to feel like anything was possible. I still had my challenges with organisation and concentration, but now I had a clever best friend and a sneaking suspicion that I might be clever too. I started doing better in class and even playing sports. To everyone's surprise, I was quite good at them. I had gone from the deep loneliness and isolation of bullying to being a part of school society. I played rugby, which was quite unbelievable to my former bullies, who were shocked that they had failed to assess my sporting potential before designating me a nerd, and it was also a shock to the girls of our year who now realised I might not be *completely* unattractive.

It lit me up. My new friend and the people he introduced me to saw me for who I really was and made me feel valuable. Adam was cool and sensitive, and he made me realise my sensitivity could be cool too. He introduced me to the idea that men having deep thoughts and feelings could be cool, even if it wasn't normal in my school or community. He had ambitions and, beside him, I realised that I could too. Our school environment was not conducive to high academic aspirations but somehow Adam and I got it into our heads that we would be a dentist and a doctor. We had both been put into the top set in the year before our GCSEs and we saw no reason why we couldn't go into academically competitive healthcare professions. It soon transpired that there was in fact one reason, and that was our rather dramatic, shared fear of needles.

In year ten, we were given our BCG jabs (a tuberculosis vaccine that is no longer part of the routine school vaccination programme) and Adam and I both very nearly fainted. I kid you not, the smart arses who were going to work in medicine nearly fainted, as a pair. It was the first look at the tools of our future trades and nearly sent us south right in front of the nurse. For many people this would be an insurmountable obstacle, but such was the confidence of our youth and the momentum we were building in our lives that it didn't feel like a problem (although our biology teacher pointed out the irony of the situation when we returned to class). We decided we simply needed some exposure therapy. So we watched YouTube videos of injections being given before gradually working up to films of surgery being performed. It actually worked – which is a good reminder of how capable we are of overcoming the blocks we may believe stand in our way. This continued the pattern of visual media facilitating my medical education, as it was only earlier that year that I had decided to become a doctor because I enjoyed watching shows about hospitals on telly. I was so taken by the confidence and capability of the doctors (actors), how they seemed to embody the poise and self-control that I lacked in my education so far, and that made them so attractive to me.

All I needed was some organisation and some drive. If I could overcome my fear of syringes, surely I could overcome my own inherent distractibility? Unfortunately, that didn't seem to be something a YouTube video would solve. I had the same challenges with focus and preparation that I always did, but now my life outside of schoolwork was more interesting than ever. Whereas in my earlier years, I had been distracted by my own mind, now I had genuine external distractions as well. Friendship, girls, going to the gym and riding a moped all seemed like far better uses of my teenage days than preparing for examinations, and for all that I knew that the exams would be central to building the life I wanted, I found it very hard to prioritise them over the immediate experiences. This is a classic challenge of executive function. I had no problem pursuing good things in the now but weighing them against greater goods in the future was nearly impossible for me.

The year of my GCSEs accelerated in the way time only does when you are having fun and, as the summer months approached, I still showed no sign of revising. Now there was the temptation to spend long days outside, fishing or playing tennis, and I reached a point where if I didn't start revising I wouldn't be going on to sixth form, let alone a medical career. My dad decided on a decisive intervention. He changed the incentives. In a moment of insight, or possibly desperation, he offered to pay me £100 for every A grade I could get in my GCSEs. This was quite a financial commitment for him: with twelve GCSEs on the horizon and a modest family income, he was at risk of paying out a significant amount. (I *really* believe my dad has ADHD and this was impulsive.) He must have considered that risk appropriate to the reward. If he ended up paying a significant sum then I would have done well, and in his mind it was worth it. Immediately, I responded. Somehow, converting the abstract idea of educational success into a pound-figure gave me a clear sense of the opportunity. Instead of hard work equalling success (which was too diffuse a concept for me), I now saw a month of solid work potentially resulting in a thousand pounds, which meant a car. Which meant freedom and adventure.

It worked. I started to cram, spending all of my days in a state of deep and dedicated concentration, working towards a finish line where a Vauxhall Corsa 1.2 SXi awaited. This was when I first discovered flow. As I studied and found my groove, hours began to pass without my noticing. The outside world became a blur as I honed in on the knowledge in front of me. Anxieties and distractions fell away and I became entirely present. Regardless of the final results, discovering that state of mind and my ability to be present were worth the effort. While examinations come and go, an understanding of our own potential is timeless, and for a young man who had doubted his ability to concentrate on anything, it was priceless.

For my dad, though, it came at the cost of over £1,000. He would argue it was the best grand he ever spent, as I did far better in my exams than anyone had predicted. I now knew I could work hard, that my seemingly shallow attention span obscured hidden depths and that I was the owner of a SXi (sexy?) Vauxhall. I was elated. My results gave me the freedom to pick the same A-level subjects as Adam and approach sixth form with the knowledge that I could apply myself.

Ideally, I would also have learned that things could be far easier if I started working just a bit earlier. However, unfortunately, that was a step too far and, as I began my A-levels, the cycle started again. It seemed as if I had to create pressure to access a state of focus, and the only way to create pressure was to leave everything until the last minute. Adam and I were cocky and we were clueless (sorry, Adam). A few days before our AS-level exams we asked our chemistry teacher whether the exams would contribute to our final A-level results. His head fell into his hands. Yes, he replied, they were half of the final grade, and the fact that we did not know this was somewhat concerning. OK, it was downright outrageous.

He was right to be concerned. For all that I tried to cram a whole year's syllabus into 36 hours, it was not enough time to save me. I learned the material, but tired myself out so much in the sleepless hours that I nearly fell asleep in the examination room. I am not exaggerating. So I had to retake that AS-level in my A-level year. Maybe it was just a clever subconscious ruse on my part to inject a bit more pressure into the process, to give me good reason, *some reason,* to finally focus.

It worked. Or, at least, it almost did. I left revision late again and this time I didn't have the added incentive of a cash prize from my dad. That wasn't a problem, though, as I now knew how satisfying studying could be and I had the clear carrot of a place at Liverpool University to study medicine if I could just get the right results. So I worked hard in the run-up to my exams, studying with the same intensity and flow that I had two years previously for my GCSEs. The exams seemed to go by without a hitch. For the first time, I felt as if my lack of executive function and inattentiveness wouldn't trip me up. But I was wrong. When the results arrived, I found that I had scored highly on my exams but fatally underperformed on a single item of coursework. My grades were close to what was required for Liverpool but even with very good exam results, I could only get a B in chemistry as my coursework had received a D grade. I look back and see how this was another step in my journey to understanding my working practices in light of my ADHD. I had learned to make myself work in the context of exam pressure but I still lacked the meticulousness to complete coursework well. You cannot cram your way out of poorly prepared coursework and I could not talk myself into Liverpool.

My headteacher did try though. She spoke at length with the admissions team at Liverpool, explaining that I had done well on every measure except for that single piece of coursework and that my failing, in that instance, had actually been the result of a misunderstanding of the brief. Unfortunately, they were not convinced but I was hugely grateful for the effort she made on my behalf.

I was deeply disappointed, but I can look back now and realise I was fortunate. As is so often the case, what I wanted was not necessarily what I needed, as the course that I did at Peninsula Medical School, based in Plymouth and Exeter, turned out to be a far better fit for me. There is a chance I would not even have completed my studies if I had been at another university. This is because Peninsula offered quite a specific approach to medical education, which fitted the quite specific nature of how I learn. While most medical courses involve long, information-heavy lectures and annual examinations, Peninsula was an outlier in how they taught and assessed us. They were a relatively new medical school and employed a very modern approach. Every two weeks, students were given a problem and a period of self-directed learning to prepare an answer to it. At the end of those two weeks, we were grilled by the lecturer on the responses we had developed. As an ADHDer, this was ideal. My own energy and attention could dictate how and when I studied, and the pressurised environment of the lecturer assessments created the conditions for my particularly dopamine-driven brain to flourish.

It was no easier than the approach at most medical universities but for me it was perfect. There was no danger of getting distracted in a long lecture and losing track of the subject. I could only move forward on any aspect of the teaching when I felt I understood it and I was able to use mixed-media methods such as video and audio learning rather than books and lectures alone. Best of all, I had a clear finish line every two weeks to work towards. I did very well and my performance was probably a stark contrast to how I would have performed in traditional medical schools, which often have five-hour lectures that I would have struggled with. In fact, I would have struggled to get past the first half hour. But at Peninsula, my hunter's brain was engaged in a pursuit every two weeks with access to all the lectures online.

My experience at Peninsula is a useful case study in how diverse education approaches can have an impact. Our learning styles are as unique as our minds and the fact that we assume education can only take one shape is often limiting. Some people excel in rigorous teaching environments and prefer rote learning, while others benefit from self-directed learning or discussion. At Peninsula, we were given room to explore and explain rather than remember and regurgitate. We still had the usual Medical School Applied Knowledge Test (MS AKT) every quarter, but in between those examinations the emphasis was on understanding and communication about the practicalities of work as a medical doctor. The approach suited me and would not necessarily be ideal for others, but I think it highlights how valuable it is to have multiple routes towards the same goals for people who learn in different ways. A more diverse learning environment would have new costs attached, particularly for personnel, but I think it would be worthwhile.

There are certain aspects of my work and education that no number of additional personnel could help me overcome, because I had to take responsibility for my own success. At university, the same issues with planning and project management that had impacted me in school continued. I regularly missed deadlines and struggled with paperwork, and I even misunderstood the submission deadline for my main essay in my final year, although I think seeing this simply as an ADHD problem may be too sympathetic, because I was old enough and capable enough to at least check the date on which I had to hand in my most important project.

It's taken me a number of years to find an approach to timelines that works for me, and I still have issues with executive function that make planning towards deadlines difficult. I've found that regular reminders about long-term projects, which fit under the banner of strategy, and short-term (daily) updates on what must be done that day works best. This keeps me clear on broader aims, with the work towards them broken down into daily tasks.

My work life now requires me to spin a lot of plates, to be conscious of many different projects across long timeframes and daily tasks that I have to deliver on time. I wouldn't be capable of doing that if I didn't have a great team around me. I took my mother's advice to hire people who are strong in the areas I am not. Whether or not you are a team leader, and however good you are (or not) with things like organisation, it is always important to be aware of the benefit of teamwork when it comes to realising your potential. We all have different perspectives and skills, and we see more and achieve more when we bring them together.

Fortunately, I have got used to hard work. Nothing is too hard if your work feels meaningful and fits with your working style. Although primary and secondary education were mostly at odds with mine, at university and in my professional life I found paths that fit around my brain. Often this was as much by chance as by design. If I had not failed to get into Liverpool I may never have experienced the style of learning that I did at Peninsula Medical School; if I had never watched *City Hospital* I might not have ended up in the ADHDers paradise (in my experience) that is A&E.

I would have loved somebody to tell me which forms of work and education would suit me best, but, as it stands, careers advice feels like an afterthought when schools are forced to focus so much on exam success. Nuanced careers advice requires deep insight and understanding of the ways in which individual young people work, but it would undoubtedly benefit anyone moving towards their professional life and our society more broadly.

We should strive for an education system that starts with wellbeing as the primary goal, both for teachers and students. This allows us to treat our outcome (well-rounded, happy individuals) and our process as one and the same, and through the creation of a happy learning environment we can get the results we want. To achieve this, we have to look at the structures in place and consider smaller class sizes, a greater number of support staff in schools and provision for mental health support across the board. This would provide greater flexibility to account for different learning styles and give teachers the time and resources to provide more tailored instruction to students who need it. For all we know, the test results, which we currently prioritise, may not improve. The evidence we have from countries that have taken approaches such as these suggest differently, though. Many of the Nordic countries do not introduce examination until well into secondary school, instead prioritising autonomy, collaboration and play, and they still outperform British schools on a number of learning measures. This points to the fact that a happy school can still be a high-achieving one.

I hope that education ministers and governments of the future see the potential our education system has. If we appreciate how our schools provide the blueprint for our society then we are duty bound to resource them and prioritise them. My work in mental health provisions and A&E has made me keenly aware of the significance of early intervention, and there is really no intervention at a societal level quite like our education system. Children should not need the luck that I had to avoid disappointing themselves. There may not always be a Mr Harris or an Adam to appear and change someone's path, but if there is an education system with the staff and resources to offer more differentiated approaches things can improve. Our outdated education system, as it stands, allows too many children to fall through the cracks.

I could have but I was lucky. I hope that my story becomes far more normal than it seems now.

4

WHY DID YOU BECOME A DOCTOR?

It takes a long time to become a doctor and even longer to truly feel like one. This is because identities take longer to learn than professions, and identities cannot be taught or examined. You must develop a mindset and manner that allows you to meet a person during the single hardest moment of their life and convey that you are the person that they most want there with them. You must learn to live with death every day and then go home for dinner. You must wake up again the next morning, put on a white coat (OK, an imaginary one – more like worn-out, poorly fitting and unflattering scrubs) and transform.

It is no wonder, then, that learning to be such a person takes a long time and unsurprising that I was so keen to become one. I had spent a large part of my youth masking, trying to build a veneer of capability and respectability to hide the small boy who felt incapable and out of place. I needed an identity strong enough to keep my inner self protected, to convince the world that there could never be someone quite so anxious or odd inside. I needed a mask, and a surgical one would do.

It is fitting that my decision to pursue medicine came out of watching *House* on television, rather than meeting any actual doctors in person.* I was drawn to people *playing doctors*, to actors who had been given the instruction to behave like a doctor and knew exactly how they were supposed to be. I wanted a role to play, and I was fortunate that the role I found gave me meaning, profound purpose and experience. Still, it could only be a mask and, like any mask, it could only protect but never cure that which it sought to hide. That would have to happen later.

Physician, heal thyself.

First, though, I had to learn to heal other people and in the early days of university, that seemed a long way off. We were thrown right in at the deep end at Peninsula Medical school, joining practising doctors and surgeons on their rounds to see the reality of the job. One of my first placements was in orthopaedic surgery and for the boy who had only a few years earlier nearly fainted at the sight of a needle, this was an eye-opener. It transpired that needles were the least of my worries – they were literally just the start of it.

In orthopaedic surgery, the tools of the trade are everything from chisels to hammers and nails, and while the work of filling a bone into shape seemed commonplace to the professionals around me,

---

*   Later, I would actually *pretend to be* Dr Gregory House when I did exams. It genuinely put me in a positive, problem-solving mindset and gave me greater self-belief. Whatever works!

it took all of my focus not to pass out. I was nineteen, watching a metal hip being slotted into a hole in someone's body, and I doubted very much whether I could ever convince anyone that this seemed normal to me. When they were done and I had not fainted, I felt a rush. I had made it through my first exposure to the reality of the medical profession and my mask hadn't slipped.

It would still be some time before we were given any actual responsibility, which was for the best. There was a lot of learning to do before lives could be put in our hands. This meant that the pressure we felt was purely academic for those first years. I would only discover how I would perform in a genuine crisis outside of the hospital. This occurred in my third year. I was driving down a dual carriageway with a friend and saw a pair of lights overtaking me on the other side of the central reservation. As soon as I realised that someone was driving on the wrong side of the road, I heard the impact, a crash that was heavier and deeper than I imagined any sound could be. We hurried to pull off at the next turning and circle back to the scene of the accident. As medical students, we hoped we could be of some use, if only to give some basic information to the real professionals when they arrived.

When we got there, the flames had died down and the two people who had been in the car that had been hit had crawled to safety. My friend went to speak with them and I turned to the elderly gentleman who had been in the car travelling the wrong way. He was in his seat, so I checked his breathing and secured his spine until the ambulance arrived. The medical teams reassured us that everyone involved in the incident was safe and should make a good recovery, and it was only once we were confident of that fact that we set off on our way.

I was so adrenalised by the experience that I had to be careful not to let my speedometer creep up to match my racing mind. I kept circling back to the fact that I had just responded to an accident and I had been calm. In fact, I had felt calmer than at almost any point in my life. The world around me had demanded my attention in a way that my brain could finally understand. I felt like I had found a place where I belonged. After so many years feeling chaotic when others were calm, I realised that I could be calm amid chaos. It had felt completely normal to me and, as strange as that may seem, it made me feel normal too. A certain comfort in high-pressure, high-octane situations is often a feature of ADHD minds and realising it could be my strength was empowering.

I had once seen my father behave in that way. There was a fight in the local Tesco and, as an off-duty police officer, he stepped into the fray. Two people were screaming and throwing punches at one another, but my father simply walked in between them and held them apart. When they had dispersed, he returned to me and continued wheeling our trolley as if nothing of note had happened. I was shaken and couldn't understand how he had the courage to step in, and the ability to walk away afterwards unfazed. I realise now that he probably has the same disposition that I do – a clarity of thought and purpose that descends when a situation becomes critical and an ability to step in and out of the mindset with ease. It is hard to describe, but the sense of clarity that a crisis provides to an often directionless and fractured mind is profound.

In A&E, these moments are heralded by the ringing of the Red Phone. This is a call from a dispatcher or ambulance that prepares the A&E team for a critical case that is arriving at their door. The voice may simply say, 'Cardiac arrest, five minutes', and the noise around you has to disappear. You have to become entirely present and all distractions must fall away. For a person with ADHD, this is like going from having fifteen tabs open on your screen to a single, critical window.

Unfortunately, this is the opposite of preparing for the multitude of examinations that you take before making it into an emergency room. Like in so many careers, the processes we use to determine someone's capability are more a test of their ability to complete examinations than they are to do the job, but I was fortunate to attend a medical school that found the middle ground. We had some written exams, which I would only ever prepare for at the last minute, but also some situational ones that were closer to the reality of being a practising doctor. You would be provided with a lifelike mannequin which would serve as your hypothetical patient. There would be monitors and charts and all the information required to treat the dummy as a real patient, while your tutors would watch and question you about what you were doing. Those tests created the perfect conditions for me to flourish. The pressure allowed me to access a hyperfocused state that I could not for my lectures or coursework, and I felt capable in a way that I never had in my education up to that point. By all accounts, that made me an odd one out. While most of my peers had always been academically successful and wanted to memorise their notes, I had to really engage with the subject matter to understand it. You could not succeed in these tests simply through diligence and preparation; you had to play a role, and that role required more autonomous learning than previously perfect students were used to.

When it came to playing the perfect academic student, I continued to struggle. Coursework was the bane of my life. I simply couldn't create the pressure around it that allowed me to focus. ADHDers chase dopamine and while a live examination is a perfect dopaminergic storm, coursework is an exercise in deferred gratification. Here's a short dopamine refresher. It is effectively a reward chemical, which is released when you achieve something hard or simply do something satisfying. It is our body's way of rewarding us for doing something good or difficult. Coursework requires you to work hard now for a pay-off later, and for people who struggle with executive function, this is an almost impossible bargain. It's a study in dopamine deferral and although that works for many people, the idea that this should be a pre-requisite for academic achievement leaves a lot of people out.

The education system has not leveraged dopamine much in our learning and testing approaches, but other fields have. Food, gaming and social media companies are deeply aware of how manipulating our dopamine responses can motivate us to eat more, play more or scroll for longer, but our education system expects us to work around our chemistry. It's an odd thing to say, but when it comes to capturing our attention and retaining it, educational resources could learn from social media feeds and some examinations would benefit from aspects of video games.

That is not to say we would want them to provide the cheap dopamine fixes those activities do. An interesting aspect of our dopamine system is that it provides greater satisfaction when the behaviour that generates it is genuinely challenging. For example, exercise breaks down chemicals that inhibit serotonin, so we feel happier from the dopamine created by a run than the that offered through a chocolate bar. So even though it is hard, we have to be aware that there isn't really such a thing as good, easy dopamine and seeking it will always cause a problem in the long term. There are risks in our reward system.

This has taken me a long time to learn and if I'm honest, I continue to grapple with my dopamine dependencies. In my personal life, easy dopamine has created more challenges for me than the hard stuff that I found at work. My time as a junior doctor included some of the most challenging days of my life but the hardest times came from my pursuit of cheap dopamine. Training as a junior doctor was fulfilling, whereas a pursuit of dopamine through food, alcohol or online validation always left me feeling empty.

There is an incredible balance of challenge and reward that comes from working in a hospital, even if the challenges are all you can really sense in the moment. My medical education took me from surgery rooms to general medicine, through A&E and obstetrics, and this gave me a chance to see what worked for me before I chose my specialism. For example, I really struggled in obstetrics. Working with mothers and babies requires a very particular skill set and, unlike in other branches of medicine, you are required to care for two people at once. I felt like a fish out of water while I was there, confident in my knowledge of medicine but without any of the experience or manner to apply it. I spent a long time feeling like an imposter, but with time began to grow more comfortable. This was the pattern across my medical training: a period of uncertainty as I entered a new domain before gaining understanding and approaches that allowed me to flourish.

I certainly struggled in the transition to postgraduate work in London because so many of the pillars of my life shifted almost immediately. I left a long-term relationship and all of my friendships in Exeter and moved to hospital accommodation in another city. I went from being a student in a relationship to a junior doctor in a single-bed room in London in a matter of days. It felt like working life, and the great city, might not be all it was cracked up to be. I am aware now that I was struggling, as I often do, with change, but I do think that my new accommodation set-up didn't help. There were a lot of different hospital staff staying there day to day and it felt like living in a very busy, derelict hotel (think peeling wallpaper, dripping taps, damp). I think anyone would find that disorientating, but I rely on having a safe home environment in which to decompress, so trying to adjust to a new city and job without that was a real challenge. It was a perfect storm of change.

I had been accepted to work in my dream hospital at Kings College London, in a city where I had always wanted to live, but I just couldn't enjoy it. Reality seemed to be catching up with my expectations everywhere that I looked. On my first weekend at Kings, I was covering the elderly care wards. There was only one senior doctor on call with me and they were stretched, so I was basically on my own. I kept looking over my shoulder for a *real* doctor who could advise me but it soon became clear that person was me, regardless of how I felt about it. My pager kept beeping and unforeseen problems kept coming up, so I was left alone to evaluate their severity and prioritise my time, which is a skill you can only learn over time. In healthcare, there are so many unknowns and so many variables when it comes to each patient's needs that you can only learn to balance them through experience. My lack of experience made that weekend feel like the busiest I ever went through on the wards, but it may simply be that I did not yet have the self-belief or knowledge to feel comfortable working through it.

It was difficult, but growth and progress often is. I felt like I had been buried under new responsibilities, but I see now that I had just been planted in new soil and these moments are what it took for me to grow. The sunshine I needed came from the other staff who came to my aid, but the nurses in particular. Some of them had thirty or forty years of experience, and they seemed to move about the place with a calmness and fluidity that I could only dream of. They were kind to me, accepted me when I became flustered and reassured me when self-doubt set in. When I became so overwhelmed that I had to ask them questions about basic medicine (like, what is the standard dose of paracetamol?) they gave me answers and reassured me that everyone is like this on their first weekend and in time I would be flying. They took care of the patients and they still found time to take care of me.

Together, we made it through that weekend and gave our patients the care they deserved, but I knew that I had to find ways to avoid becoming overwhelmed. I could be calm in a crisis, but I couldn't keep feeling like I was having a crisis when everyone else seemed calm. It was not a simple problem to solve, though. I couldn't simply make myself a confident doctor overnight, but I could take steps to go easier on myself. I had to look at my situation and try to gain perspective that kept me from catastrophising. *I am a junior doctor,* I told myself, *I am learning and I am not perfect yet. The only thing that will keep me from improving is ruminating on being inadequate, so I have to accept where I am, do my best and try to improve.*

When we suffer with imposter syndrome, we are often setting unattainable standards for ourselves, comparing our own performance with elite performers or those who are far further along in their journey. I had to be realistic, to manage my expectations and believe in all the evidence that said I was operating at a reasonable level. With that mindset, and with time, I started to grow more confident and gained the experience I needed to be able to balance the priorities of patient care.

Evaluating patient needs against one another and organising your time accordingly is a huge part of being a doctor; alongside medical knowledge and bedside manner, it forms the key components of the profession. I had the knowledge and I was good with people, but my lack of executive function made organising and planning my time the area in which I had to improve. So I watched others and I learned. I studied the nurses and senior doctors around me and how they prioritised their time and I took it on board. Gradually, I improved. I learned how to differentiate the most pressing needs from those that could be delegated or seen to later, but also learned that if I trusted my instincts and ability, I could free up my mind to make good decisions. I found ways to be productive that built on an understanding of my own ways of working and some of the idiosyncrasies of my own mind. For example, we would do a ward round each morning with a senior doctor and then set out a list of tasks to be completed that day. Once I had my list, I would order them in terms of priority and set points where I would earn a break and a treat (a snack or a coffee). So I would know that once I had done five of my fifteen tasks I'd have an americano, eight tasks and I'd have lunch and after twelve tasks I'd stop for a banana. It sounds small but by introducing these rewards mindfully, I gave myself access to dopamine rather than continued slow progress.

It also allowed me to focus on what I had to do in manageable components, rather than grow anxious at the sheer scale of the totality of jobs to do. This saved me from the negative cycle of worry and self-criticism, which was integral to staying happy and productive. We all find it difficult to plan if we are panicking and no one can dedicate their whole mind to a problem if much of it is focused on self-criticism.

The mental and physical strains that are part of the medical profession forced me to learn endurance and cultivate consistency in changing conditions. No two days on a ward are the same and nights are another space entirely. As a junior doctor, I did not take care of my mind or body, which made adapting difficult. I would work, long hard weeks (sometimes in twelve-day stretches) and then 'recharge' by going to the pub over the weekend, which only led me to feel worse when I returned on Monday. I lived unhealthily while doing a job that can put a strain on your health, which would have been hard enough without the regularly changing shift patterns.

At some points, I would work days and then switch over to evenings and then nights. As a person with (undiagnosed) ADHD, this required a lot of adaptation. I found myself unable to sleep through the days, turning up to work unrested, or I could return home from a night shift in the morning light with too much adrenaline to bed down for the day. Unsurprisingly, it impacted my cognitive function.

All humans struggle to perform well without adequate sleep and for people with ADHD this is particularly pronounced. Shift work is a challenge to our bodies and brains, and studies show that the risk of certain cancers rises 3.3 per cent for every five years of shift work and depressive symptoms by 33 per cent. I had to learn to adjust, but I'm glad to say that NHS trusts have become more conscious of the needs of shift workers. Hospitals try not to make people work too many night shifts in a row and offer leniency for neurodivergent people who are so dependent on their sleep schedules.

After spending my first year as a doctor at King's College Hospital, I moved to Lewisham Hospital, where I continued to work throughout my years in clinical practice. Lewisham Hospital was full of amazing people, and getting to know them changed me as a doctor and as a person. I arrived at the A&E department there with some experience but I still felt like a bit of an impostor. I had grown more comfortable in my role and I knew that I had the knowledge to perform well, but any time that I didn't I would blame myself, falling into a loop of self-criticism. The problem was that I was now a doctor and how I performed in my job could be the difference between life and death, so self-criticism seemed more valid than ever. I was a perfectionist in a job where perfection was impossible to achieve.

The fundamental reality is that you cannot get it right all the time, and you cannot 'save' everyone. You should always strive for excellence in medicine, but never expect perfection. My perfectionism was tied to a sense that I needed to be perfect to even be *good enough*. This is a vicious cycle in a high-stakes and high-pressure environment like A&E. Doctors have to accept that we are not infallible and that we could make mistakes with terrible consequences in our pursuit of positive outcomes. Our job is to limit the mistakes, learn when they happen and try to give the best care we can in every situation. As one consultant once told me, any doctor who says they have never made a mistake is either not being truthful or hasn't worked long enough. This can be a hard thing to accept when you are working in such a demanding and life-changing profession, but if you do not you risk entering into a negative spiral of self-criticism and poor performance.

I worked my way out of those negative spirals of thought with the help of my colleagues and mentors. One in particular came into my life when I most needed it and has continued to be there for me in the years since. I met him in my first year of A&E medicine and I immediately realised that he was the sort of doctor I wanted to be. He was deeply experienced but chose to earn respect rather than demand it. He stood at the top of a hierarchy but spoke with junior doctors and patients alike as equals. He remained calm even when the circumstances around him were fraught and tensions grew. I was desperate to learn how he did it and after some time, I plucked up the courage to ask how he remained unfazed by the swirling complexities that surrounded us, and kept his head after so many years experiencing the highs and lows of an A&E department.

His answer was as much philosophy as it was professional advice and although I can't recall his words precisely, his sentiment has crystallised into the following principles that I take forward in my life to this day:*

Control that which you can control. We have been conditioned to believe that, ideally, in any profession, we would be in complete control of everything, but this is simply impossible. We have to understand that there are many things in our professional and daily lives that we cannot control, and accept them. Only then are we able to work on the very real problems we have.

Do your best and forgive yourself when your best is not enough. Our meritocratic society teaches us that we can always do better and be better, but in reality, our effort is all we can really control. We should focus on doing our best because there is nothing more that we can do.

Know that you will not be able to save everyone. Even the perfect course of action will not always be enough. In medicine, as in life, we

---

* In fact, much of it may be wisdom I collected from him and others at different points – memory is funny like that.

can do the same thing in ten situations and see ten different results. So we must accept our limitations.

Take pride in your work but do not take your failures personally. Because energy spent criticising yourself is energy you are not using to help the next person.

You must take care of yourself if you are going to be able to take care of somebody else. Because you are no use to anyone if you are burned out.

It takes a smart person to hold wisdom like that, but a kind one to offer it to their struggling junior halfway through a night shift, which I think is the sort of person that A&E medicine attracts. But these are also the things that working in such a department teaches us. In hospitals, and in A&E in particular, we can't help but be reminded, every day, that we will all die. I believe that the messages above, about accepting a lack of control and our limitations, are inextricably linked to this appreciation of our mortality. Doctors have to accept that we are only human, and we are reminded of our fallibility and our mortality more often than most.

This constant reminder, that life is imperfect, precious and vulnerable, is humbling but it is also *enlivening*. They say you never know what you have got till it's gone and in some ways, being closer to death and the dying gave me a sense of quite how incredible it is to be alive. I think we fail to appreciate how special that is. We treat living like it is *normal,* we take it for granted and act like we are here forever. If there is a norm to unpick from this, it would be that we have normalised acting like we will live forever or get another go. We will not. Life is short, it is precious and is liable to be ended by things that we could never see coming. If we can remember this, we can appreciate it. In billions of years of history, you are alive for this short window, *now*. If that is not worth appreciating, what is? Try to remind yourself of that every day, just as I was reminded of it each morning when I left the hospital and each night when I returned.

There were times, of course, when I didn't think I could last another night in A&E. It takes a great deal of grit to endure the difficulties that A&E presents, as well as wisdom that I did not always have to overcome the challenges. That certainly felt the case on Christmas Eve 2017. It had been one of those gruelling night shifts when everything that could go wrong did, and everyone who could usually do something about it couldn't. In an attempt to take care of myself before effectively taking care of everybody else, I decided to take a breather in an equipment cupboard beside the A&E waiting room. This wasn't something I did often but it was Christmas, everywhere else was full and I needed a moment. So I sat with my head in my hands and repeated the sort of things that I always told myself in these situations. *You can do this. You are a good doctor. Breathe.*

As I began to breathe, a wild banging reverberated through the stockroom door and a man's voice shouted across the divide. 'I've been here for hours. Why haven't I been seen yet? I know you're in there!' It was a patient who had become tired of waiting and decided that the junior doctor in the cupboard was the best person to solve his problem. He didn't want to spend his Christmas in A&E and neither did I. So I kept hiding and pondered whether this was in fact the lowest moment in my career. It was as if Christmas had crystallised the reality of the situation. Our service was understaffed and under-resourced, and the man outside felt like the representative of a society that thought my colleagues and I were responsible for that fact. Of course, we were not, but we were responsible for delivering care and I knew that I could face up to it, so after a few more deep breaths, I returned to the ward and reassured the gentleman that we would do our best to see him.

It is only when I look back on these moments, and my career since leaving A&E, that I truly understand the meaning of 'control that which you can control'. While I was working as a doctor, I always thought my colleague meant that we should focus on the medical care we could give instead of worrying about that which we could not, but now I see it differently. I see that his logic applied to my situation that night and my frustration with the whole medical system in which I worked. I could not control the successive governments who had failed to fund our service or train the staff we needed. I could not control a society that fails to treat mental and physical wellbeing until people end up in Accident and Emergency rooms. I could not make that man on the other side of the stock-room door that Christmas morning see that I was as disappointed by the situation as he was. I was a doctor, not a policymaker, so it was my job to heal people's bodies not change people's minds. I could only control that which I could control.

Which may be why, via an incredibly circuitous and fortuitous route, I became someone who talked about healthcare and policy, rather than someone who delivered it. On some level, I must have realised that controlling that which I could control, in a system that felt out of control, would not always be right for me. I realised that the accidents and the emergencies we treated began far away from the rooms in which we delivered care because sickness began in schools, workplaces and Government offices. If I could not help people consider what happens in our pubs, what's on our plates and the things that affect our personal lives, I would do nothing to stop problems being passed down to A&E departments. I would not stop junior doctors in broom cupboards being blamed when those departments could not treat all of society's ills. I had to try to normalise new ways of living that made people well because we had reached a point where we could not deal with the number who are sick.

If you want to understand the unifying idea behind this book, it is just that. I want to explain how I have become more understanding of myself, how we can be more understanding of one another and in the process rethink the norms that determine how we all live. Because in thinking about my problems, I have had to think about what we normalise at a societal level and the problems we push to the doors of Accident and Emergency rooms by ignoring them. We must relieve the pressure on our healthcare services by making our society healthier and we must support those services to help people who are sick. There's a long way to go, but I'd like to use my experience to think about what we can do for hospitals now.

We must truly appreciate people who dedicate their lives to the care of others in hospitals. This involves paying them well, giving them a manageable workload and providing the resources and training they need to do their job properly. We have seen medical staff of all stripes requesting improved pay and working conditions over the last few years, and I think they reflect differences in perspective that will not be resolved through a single pay agreement. These are clearly questions of what we value as a society, as the well-publicised tensions in the medical profession have been echoed by emergency service professionals across the board. Members of the police, military and fire services have all said similar things. A society that does not appreciate its emergency workers is a society that will fail.

We need to stop applying the logic of business to healthcare because it simply does not work. Private contractors and management consultants will never be able to evaluate and improve a public service like medicine because it is not a field where you are evaluated by profit and loss. Our performance is defined by the health and sickness of the people we care for. You will never see a private contractor bidding for the right to run A&E departments because they are incredibly expensive, dangerous environments. Any attempt to find marginal financial gains in these areas will result in loss of life. We can either provide more funds to A&E or we can fund mental health, social services and elderly care to cut down the number of people arriving there, but we cannot consult our way out of this reality.

We should have more staff, more doctors in senior management roles and more flexibility in the working environment. Medicine is a vocational career and as a result staff, have been willing to accept that they are neither treated nor paid as well as their peers in other fields that require a similar education level, but vocation may soon no longer be enough.

Finally, we need to think more deeply about where, when and why our health services are engaged. Currently, we have a healthcare system that has normalised curing sickness rather than promoting health and therefore it mostly kicks into action when people become ill. My experience has shown me this is a vital service, but I believe we need to think more about promoting wellbeing outside of the hospital doors. A&E is a crucial last resort but what is the first?

One area may be in the provision of more access to fitness and wellbeing support outside of hospital. GPs can currently prescribe things like membership to fitness centres and personal trainers, and I think this is a great start. We should look at encouraging a population that is fitter, stronger through later life and able to join in group exercise activities. There are numerous benefits to these more proactive solutions, but we can be confident that such efforts would reduce stress on our healthcare system. For example, muscle mass is often described as a longevity indicator in older populations because strength and stability protect us from falls and injuries in later life. Our hospitals spend a lot of time treating older people who have suffered injuries that they may have been able to avoid if they had access to some strength training, so this would be a step to protecting people and reducing the load on emergency services.

We would also benefit from the psycho–social impacts that sport- and wellbeing-focused interventions would confer. Another norm that has been internalised in healthcare is a sort of 'dualism' – the idea that the mind and body are distinct entities that don't really impact one another. I passionately believe that we need to consider provisions that promote mental fitness and wellbeing (physical training is only one of these) because they will help people live more happily and avoid the numerous physical conditions connected to mental health challenges, which range from cardiovascular conditions to cancers and degenerative conditions like Alzheimer's. The more we can think about mental fitness as a guard against physical sickness in the long run, the better able we will be to create a healthcare system that not only cures illness but protects against it.

Establishing a new norm of healthcare is my greatest passion and the focus of most of my work today. If we can think of healthcare as health promotion and understand mental fitness as a driver of physical health then we will have made great strides toward creating a healthier society and a better NHS. It may take time but progress often does.

I once treated an incredible woman who had a few weeks to live. Her life had been hard – at every turn, she had faced ill health and the loss of those closest to her. After getting to know her, I asked her for the secret of her happiness, because she always seemed to be smiling. She told me that as long as she was alive, she would smile, because to be alive was her greatest privilege. I realised it was mine too, and that my second greatest privilege was to learn from someone like her during the last weeks of her life, because it was people like her who had made me into a doctor.

Moreover, she helped me to appreciate just how special it is to be alive. It is rare, it is wonderful and it is something to smile about. Dying people taught me that. And I am so grateful to have had access to that wisdom before my life too comes to end. We must normalise the appreciation of being alive. This means, like A&E doctors the world over, engaging with the reality that we will all die. Whether this means helping others who are grieving or supporting people who are in the process of passing on will depend on your approach and situation, but we can no longer try to keep death at arm's length, out of society's view. Then we must practise gratitude – not for the 'great' things, the lottery wins and the perfect days, but for the simple fact of being alive.

I know that one day I will be in the position that my smiling patient was too. I hope that, like her, I will have taught someone else to smile. I also hope that I will have a doctor or nurse beside me, and that they will know how much I appreciate them.

5

HOW IS YOUR LOVE LIFE?

Self-awareness is arguably more important in love and relationships than in any other aspect of our lives. When we commit to partnerships with other people, we combine our hopes and fears, and our gifts and limitations, to create something singular. This means that our relationships are only as strong as our understanding of our part in it, and as enduring as our ability to communicate how we feel about ourselves and what we have built together. Our job in a relationship is to try to understand ourselves and the other person, and to find paths through life that allow us both to feel valued.

Unfortunately, the details of my intimate relationships are to be considered part of my job because I was once a reality TV contestant. I was in a game show about love, which is a strange state of affairs, and one that puts your love affairs in a strange state. When you have been on a show like *Love Island*, anyone you are involved with romantically before or afterwards becomes a public figure by association, which is unfair on them. While I chose to become a public figure (somewhat accidentally, as we will see), to respect privacy, I'm not going to talk about my past relationships and instead focus on core themes that relate to ideas of normality in this area. So I'll approach romantic relationships through the lens that we all experience them – beginnings, middles and ends.

The romantic norm about the beginning of a relationship is that we should fall hard and fast. It is almost as if we believe that, like an atom bomb, all the potential energy of a lasting love should be compressed into that initial excitement of a first meeting. There's an idea that we should *know* when we have found someone we can build a relationship with. But I think this is open to evaluation. In my view, complex people, like all complex things, take time to understand and the excitement of a first meeting may not be a sign of enduring compatibility. In fact, it may not even be related. Excitement is a feature of the unknown and it is only in knowing others that we can develop the understanding required to achieve compromises and to support each other.

Although we should go into relationships with an open mind, we must practise self-awareness and try to be conscious of falling hard and fast. Falling in love is a chemical overload – our brains are flushed with serotonin and oxytocin – and this has a tendency to make us think in ways that we would not normally. The very normal tendency to start imagining possible futures with someone we hardly know in the present may be enjoyable, but it opens us up to a greater sense of loss when our expectations or hopes are not met.

Love doesn't need us to be pessimists, and maybe we don't even need to be realists, but it's always helpful to avoid becoming a fantasist.

This is not selfishness and, in fact, keeping our expectations in check is something we can do for our partners, as well as ourselves. There's nothing worse than feeling like someone really appreciates you and then watching as their fantastical view of you gradually diminishes with experience. It makes you feel as if the reality of you is a problem, when in fact it is the fantasy of you that was always the issue. This is something that we all need to be conscious of because a misunderstanding of it underlies popular current ideas in love and dating, like 'the ick'. Our date may struggle to close an umbrella or tie their shoelaces and the spell gets broken. The fact that such small things can serve to make someone unattractive is not just a testament to how fragile that attraction is but also how it depends on an imaginary ideal of someone. Only a perfect person could close every umbrella they ever hold with total swiftness and grace, and perfect people do not exist. If we build others up with our own imaginations, the reality of their normality will never come close and we will always eventually find something that doesn't meet our expectations. It is only by giving other people time and aligning our view of them to a growing set of shared experiences that we can have any consistency or durability in our impression of them. Anything else is careless.

So we need to appreciate just how much the early days of getting to know another person is a time of great vulnerability for both ourselves and others. This is essential because a certain amount of vulnerability is baked into the start of any relationship.

The first months of any love involve the peeling away of our defence mechanisms and the presentation of deeper, more intimate parts of ourselves. We start by offering the version of ourselves that we present to the world (or worse, the one that we present to an app) and gradually let someone get closer to the one that we are inside. We introduce someone to our insecurities and our oddities, and by revealing these things that we hide from the rest of the world, we grow intimate.

As someone who has engaged in a form of masking all my life, this is a challenge. So much of what I have tried to do through school and my professional life has involved creating the image of a normal, capable man, which kept others from seeing the reality underneath. If your internal reality is so opposed to your external presentation, it can be hard to bridge the gap when someone initially falls for the person that you present to the outside world. This has made it a struggle to accept the vulnerability that comes with intimacy. We all mask and we all hide vulnerability, so the more we can understand and appreciate those parts of ourselves we consider true, core values, the less vulnerable we will feel when we gradually remove our masks.

This fear, of being unmasked and unacceptable, may explain the rejection sensitivity that many people feel. We often have to build up so many defences that we are hypersensitive when we let people pass them. When you have gone to such lengths to protect the real you from criticism, you are particularly hurt when that criticism does come. We need to develop a core sense of worth that allows us to receive feedback from people we trust, or any reaction that is less than completely positive will feel like stinging criticisms that cut to the quick and we react defensively.

If we lack an appreciation of ourselves then there is a risk that we see criticism as a reflection of reality, that a person we love is confirming something we already believe – that we are not enough. People who feel this way, who believe that they are not worthy of love, think others will see it too and will push them away. This is evidently self-defeating and yet so hard to stop. When a loved one criticises us within a partnership (within reason), we should ideally be able to take it as given that they are doing so while remaining committed to pursuing that partnership. That when someone suggests changes or compromises in our behaviour they are doing so because they want a future for us both.

In fact, I think working on ourselves means accepting that we are more than the fixed entity that exists in our self-critical imaginations. It is because many of us start from a place of self-doubt, a belief that we actually couldn't be better, that we take offence at the suggestion that we could be different. If we have a low opinion of ourselves it extends to doubting our ability to improve, and this makes having a changing, growing relationship a hard thing.

It is equally important to have a sense of our intrinsic value when it comes to conflict, which is a normal part of any relationship, romantic or otherwise. Many of us tend to see conflict as a result of some problem with ourselves or another person, rather than an issue that has arisen from a certain context or instance. This is not a healthy way to approach it. It's always more productive to discuss behaviour that we find problematic in terms of how it makes us feel rather than through a more absolute statement about the other person. For example, the statement 'I feel a bit scared when you drive so quickly' is completely different to 'You are a careless driver'; 'I feel disappointed that you forgot about our dinner date' is not the same as telling someone 'you are so thoughtless'. At the same time, if we internally convert statements about how someone feels into reflections of who we are, then even the most sensitive discussion of preferences or differences in opinion can feel the same as a personal attack.

So we must value ourselves if we are to value our relationships. Only then can we find the compromises and balance that allow us to progress past those early days when we are discovering another person's boundaries to the point where we are planning a future together. Communication is key. Our modern world has normalised quite limited communication and the internet in particular has changed how we interact. On the internet, people are either showing or telling, and more often than not they are arguing. There is very little room for understanding.

In contrast, as much as possible, communication in relationships should be built around listening to what another person really feels and to our own feelings. When people build a partnership, they share both their strengths and their vulnerabilities, and, as such, it is vital that we listen to one another without prejudice. Sometimes, we may even need to listen to the feelings beneath a partner's words. This can be difficult, and it takes practice, but emotional intelligence is something we can learn. When our partner tells us that they don't want to do something, we can either consider this as a reflection of their unwillingness to support us in something we want to do or as a reflection of some vulnerability they may not have been able to put into words yet. Maybe they are scared, maybe experiences they had in their past make a reasonable and normal thing (to you) seem difficult. Our role is to understand the people we love in such a way that we can help them understand themselves, and often this means giving them not only the benefit of the doubt but the benefit of insight.

This insight can only come from true, mutual understanding. As much as possible, we should discuss our hopes and fears with the people we love (romantically or otherwise) and understand what makes the former hopeful and the latter fearful. This can only be built on self-knowledge. If we don't know what we want, what a happy life or progress looks and feels like to us, there is no way we can communicate it to another person. We must value and understand ourselves if we are to value someone else, because without that, we will be too vulnerable and too uncertain to build and plan.

This takes time – both with ourselves and with other people – but taking time is not something we normalise in our society today. There is a paradox of choice when it comes to relationships that means many people feel like there is always another option. This is where more choice can be a good thing, but too many choices can become distressing or unsatisfying. Take the example of a trip to the shops: you may prefer to have a choice between two types of orange juice rather than just one, you may even like the idea of three, but if you are offered forty different options, the choice becomes overwhelming. At a certain point, you feel that no matter which you choose, there may have been another, better orange juice that you failed to find. The paradox of choice points to the fact that in a field of many options, we are more likely to focus on what we have not chosen than feel satisfied with what we have.

The contemporary world of dating apps may have created one of the most dissatisfying and paradoxical choice environments imaginable. There are now more potential partners available than ever, one dopamine-laden swipe away, but people seem less satisfied by dating than they once did. In part, this is because the investment people are willing to make in any one relationship is reduced because there is a sense that many others are available, but also because the effort that is required is quite limited. Whereas once, meeting someone and agreeing on mutual attraction required some bravery and conversation, now it is greenlit by a tech company. While it used to take some work, and a good deal of validation, to find out that someone might be interested in a date, now it can come with very little input and the resulting sense that it is not as meaningful. Furthermore, that lack of effort to get to the starting point of a relationship is reflected in the effort people are willing to put in to get to know another person.

We have all met someone – a friend, colleague or partner – who we didn't much like at first but who we've grown to have a satisfying relationship with in time. Maybe we were required to spend more time together by circumstance and gradually came to recognise the things that we shared and aspects of their outlook that we liked, and we had experiences together that bonded us. In an online world where new matches are almost infinitely and immediately available, the likelihood of taking such time is reduced. Just as fast fashion may leave us with many clothes we do not wear, so does rapid online dating leave us with many matches we do not really appreciate. Making a connection is not always immediate, but the immediacy of our modern world and dating in particular means connection is harder than ever to find.

It also encourages superficiality. While most of us will factor appearance into our choice of a partner, the new normal asks us to make a snap judgement based not only on their physical appearance in a few photos, but how their professional, social and personal life come across on a page. I think this has occurred alongside the growth of social media, which has normalised judgement of people based on an image that they cultivate for the internet rather than their true self. In turn, people idealise lifestyles and personalities that are glorified by the internet, and revere those who look like Instagram models and behave like wealth-influencers. Young people increasingly expect their partners to be rich and beautiful, sharing those things on the internet, when the foundations of a durable love have nothing to do with money or appearance. Love is private and it takes time: we would all do well to remind ourselves of that.

If we can take our time, we may find someone we want to spend more time with. If, as we get to know someone, we can practise the self-understanding and empathy that facilitates compromise and forward planning then we may start to build a life together. Though, of course, we may do all of these things and realise that we are simply not compatible. This is nothing to be ashamed of – relationships end and it doesn't always have to be one person or another's fault.

As much as possible, we should strive to see the end of a relationship as a circumstance rather than a reflection of some problem with our self or another person. We all fear rejection and it can be hard not to treat a break-up as a rejection of ourselves. But it need not be. A break-up is what happens when two people have come to recognise that a partnership is not in their best interests, but we can remain confident that we are still as worthy of love as ever.

The end of a loving relationship is a challenging time for our sense of self-worth, and the more secure it is generally the better we will be able to navigate the hurt that comes with breaking up. If we have a fragile sense of self-worth, a core belief that at a deeper level, we are probably not worthy of love, a break-up can feel like a confirmation of that. We have to cultivate self-compassion before we can build lasting love or successfully negotiate out of a love that has run its course. This is the only way to ensure that we can love well and are able to forgive ourselves when loving relationships come to an end.

Self-compassion is not self-esteem and it is not selfishness. Trying to be compassionate to ourselves does not mean ignoring our mistakes or trying to be better, but understanding that all people have a value simply in virtue of being, and that our value is not compromised by mistakes or failures. It can be very hard to practise self-compassion when we are struggling with a break-up. Our first step is to separate our sense of value from the relationship that has ended. If we can focus on our core values, which existed before a relationship started and which will endure throughout our lives, then we have a secure and consistent foundation upon which to start building. We should also try to practise focusing on the things we appreciate about ourselves rather than fixating on what we've done wrong. All of us have traits, actions and behaviours to be proud of, and if we can remind ourselves of them, we can see that they are independent of the outcome of any one romantic relationship. This is an important practice for developing self-compassion at any time in our lives, but it is vitally important when a relationship comes to an end. At these times, we must connect with ourselves through kindness, rather than be cruel to ourselves or avoidant.

Avoidance, at any difficult time in my life, often took the form of dependence on food or alcohol. Many of us seek something outside of ourselves that we can attach to when we are not happy in ourselves or our present, but these dependencies rarely help us to grow happier. It is only by sitting with ourselves and getting to know and value the person we are that we can begin creating a new future. At some point, in any journey where there is loss, we come to understand it and ourselves better, and it is then that we are able to progress more happily.

Significant life changes present different challenges depending on the stage of our lives in which we find ourselves, but improved self-knowledge and compassion is always a good remedy. When we are older, the end of a relationship can feel deeply alienating because we have become so used to living in a partnership or feel our capacity for growth is limited. When we are younger, we have simply not had the time to get to know ourselves and develop a belief in our ability to grow. It is only by sitting with ourselves, at any age, that we will be able to determine who we are *now* and make decisions about what would make that person happy.

I say this as someone who arrived in their thirties without taking enough time to understand himself and who experienced both good and bad things as a result. I've already talked about many of the difficulties that I encountered as a result of a lack of self-knowledge, but it is clear to me that there are many things in my life that I might not have pursued if I were as self-aware as I am now. I may never have ended up in the position that I am, speaking to you, and I certainly wouldn't have gone on reality television.

People don't believe me when I tell them how naive I was going into *Love Island*. I had just finished a residency at Lewisham Hospital and got approached on a dating app to appear on the show. I wasn't sure it was for me but one of the consultants I worked with suggested that I should at least go down to the casting interview for a laugh. I didn't take it very seriously and never expected to hear anything back from the team who make the show, so you can imagine my surprise when they asked me to make travel plans. I weighed it up for a few hours and then decided, somewhat impulsively, that it could be fun. Having finished my residency at Lewisham Hospital, it seemed like a good time to take a break, so I figured it could be a good way to get a free holiday and then return to A&E with a tan and a few funny stories. I had no idea it could change my life.

In fact, *Love Island* completely changed my identity, even though it did not change who I was at my core. I had grown secure in the idea of myself as an A&E doctor and was very happy and content in my life, but as soon as I stepped through the doors of the villa, I knew that this identity and the safety I found in it was gone. I was nervous and felt naked, which was fitting because we were all mostly almost naked anyway. On the first day, I arrived and waited in a green room for a few hours. My anxiety ratcheted up and I decided that I was going to be rejected in some form. This was both a sort of paranoia and a reasonable prediction of what would follow because I was rejected. I didn't fit the ideal of a *Love Island* man – I was a pale non-bodybuilder, which in the real world doesn't look odd, but in those circumstances, it made me look pretty peculiar. I wasn't someone who had ever thought of love as a game, and I didn't draw meaning or any part of my identity from my ability to attract other people. I wasn't good at *Love Island* and, in truth, I know now that the sort of self-awareness, empathy and kindness that are pre-conditions for love have nothing to do with entertainment television.

Since my ADHD diagnosis I have focused, in all areas of my life, on knowing myself and loving myself. So many of the difficulties we experience stem from a fear of intimacy and of letting another person see the truth of us that we have learned to mask. Like everyone, I need to accept vulnerability because it is a precondition for love, and I have to continue to adapt as my life changes and I do too. It may be hard but truly good things are rarely easy, and if love and learning can blossom alongside one another then I am happy to do the work.

We can say that loneliness creates hardship and that connection breeds joy, but there is no reason to pre-suppose that the most meaningful and joyful life for any one person *should* centre on a romantic attachment. In the same way, we should not assume that marriage and having children is the best path for all of us. Women in particular are ostracised for choosing not to have children, or for living alone. Our norms presuppose that parenthood and marriage are the right path for everyone – and this denies the individuality and uniqueness of any one person's circumstances. We should be conscious of the pressure we put on ourselves and one another to live lives and maintain relationships that meet the standards of our norms. It is much more effective, and joyful, to realise what kind of connection gives us meaning and what works for us. Many people do not find joy in their romantic relationships and they should be free to end them, just as people who are happy without a romantic partnership should not feel pressure to enter one. We should take time to know ourselves and, with that knowledge, decide what is best for us. The alternative is living less happily, blinkered by norms and stuck in a limited view of our own self and happiness.

6

ARE YOU LONELY?

Ever since I was a child, I've sought the safety of my own company when the social world has not seemed to be a peaceful place. The challenge has always been to re-emerge. Learning about why I retreat and how I foster connections again is an ongoing process for me. I'm still learning that the fears that keep me isolated are not insurmountable and beginning to accept that a certain amount of discomfort is necessary to overcome them. In the long term, I know that the difficulty of facing my fears is nothing compared to the sadness of living beneath them, even if the passive choice often seems easier in the short term.

Growing up, I was often governed by my fears and regularly unhappy because of it. I had some friendships as a younger child but there were many times when my fear of rejection or tendency to catastrophise kept me from enjoying my social life. I rarely had a birthday party as a child because I worried that no one would attend. In this case, my fears were self-fulfilling because I gave them too much respect. My fear that people would not want to come to my parties meant that I would not invite them. I missed out on joy because of a fear of some hypothetical pain.

I always struggled to take my friendships outside of my school's four walls. I didn't like to let people into my space, and for a long time, I felt anxious at the prospect of inviting friends into my home. I couldn't yet see that my fear of the worst-case scenario *was* the worst-case scenario, because there is nothing more frightening than a life lived – or not lived – in fear.

As I grew older, I became better at making friends and entering into new spaces with them, but the fear of the unknown persisted. I knew the games I wanted to play and the social life that I wanted to have, but for a long time, my anxiety around engaging still overrode my motivation. I desperately wanted to join sports teams as a young teenager, but my ability to catastrophise meant that as I grew closer to making the leap, the hurdles only seemed to grow. I would agree to join a practice session or a match, but, in the days before, I would become so consumed with abstract fears that I would conclude that it was not worth the trouble. I think, ultimately, that I was afraid of rejection or shame. When I look back, my overriding fear was of not being picked or being seen as unworthy of involvement. At its core, my low self-image made me afraid that by *trying,* my fears about myself would be confirmed. It was only through the support of friends and the new perspectives they provided that I ever over-came my fear and the dragging weight of low self-esteem.

In my late teens, my friend Sam helped me do just that when he suggested I join a training session at a local rugby club. I circled around the familiar drain of anxiety and the isolation of my own thoughts, but he kept pulling me back, reminding me that the session would be fun and that he would be there with me. After a week of catastrophising and very nearly pulling out, and a car journey spent sick with worry, it only took ten minutes of play for me to know that I loved the experience. There was nothing to be afraid of, but it made such a difference to have someone beside me to help me realise that. This is the power of friendship but also a reflection of the pernicious nature of loneliness. We grow lonely in part because of our fears, but in our loneliness, we only become more fearful. We often need a helping hand if we are to break out of that cycle, and yet helping hands can be harder to grasp when we have distanced ourselves from others.

I struggled with isolation when I left *Love Island*. I retreated from the world because I saw it as a hostile place that I lacked the resources to deal with, which was not entirely a product of my imagination. I had become a public figure and I was really *not* prepared for it. I went into *Love Island* thinking of it as no more than a holiday and a few funny stories, never expecting much to change in my life. When I told the other contestants that, they laughed: to them, I was naive and set for a rude awakening. While to my eyes, they had a distorted view of how much the show meant to people and they were overly optimistic about how it could transform our lives.

I gradually realised that it was me who was probably wrong when new contestants arrived from the outside and told me off camera about how my profile had grown. They informed me that I already had a few hundred thousand followers on Instagram, which I thought impossible, given my account was set to private. Another contestant explained that it had been switched to a public account and received a blue tick, verifying me as a public figure. This is a good metaphor for what was happening to me more broadly: I was being made into a public figure whether I wanted it or not.

I failed to appreciate how my world was changing and how lonely that could make me, but I don't blame myself. It was a rapid, disorientating transformation, taking place in a world that I had been cut off from. I had arrived in Spain, handed in my phone and spent a few nights in isolation with a chaperone before entering the hermetically sealed box of the show, and it was outside of that space, beyond my view, that the world changed in its attitude to me. This is a peculiar thing to experience and something that has rarely occurred outside of a very specific moment in the twenty-first century. When before had someone disconnected from the world and become incredibly visible to it in the process? Or got on a plane as a doctor and come back as a sort of celebrity?

In the final days of the programme, the producers tried to make us aware of what to expect back in the real world. They explained that the viewing figures had been very high and that we should expect a fair bit of attention, but I lacked the imagination to really understand what that meant. It was only when I landed in London that I started to sense how much had changed. On my first day back, my friend Sam and I went into town to replace my phone, which had died under the weight of WhatsApp and Instagram notifications. He said it was best that we didn't travel there by tube because we would probably get hassled. I didn't believe him and I couldn't justify a taxi, so we took the tube anyway.

I realised my mistake very quickly. At Oxford Circus station, we struggled to leave the train because we were surrounded by people taking selfies and when we finally reached the Apple store on Regent Street, the crowd followed us in. The commotion was so great that the staff served us separately and pushed us out of their store to calm things down. It was odd – people weren't motivated to photograph me because they liked my work or respected me, but because they wanted a photo to show that I existed in the real world, rather than just on their television screen. It felt like they wanted proof that I wore something other than swimming trunks and brightly coloured shirts, had conversations about something other than 'coupling up' and did things like ride the tube.

People feel a certain kind of ownership of 'characters' from reality TV. We are ordinary people who have become recognisable simply through being watched, who lack the professional credentials of actors or musicians, and it means we also lack a certain distance from the audience. I was famous for being seen on television and now people were exercising their right to see me in the real world.

For six months, things continued on that track. Increasingly, I felt like an exotic bird that was there to be caught in the trap of a selfie, and I really didn't enjoy it. Don't get me wrong – I appreciated the love and support I received, but fame itself isn't that easy. While other people assumed I must be having a great time, dining out on my recognition and becoming rich in the process, I was doing none of that. I didn't want to do nightclub appearances and I had no clue how to do adverts, so I remained stuck – too famous for the tube and too broke to take a taxi. For my mental health and for my bank balance, I decided to go back to A&E. That was the first time I felt a sense of normality again and some respite from the loneliness I was experiencing. I was able to put on my doctor's costume for a few months and return to a version of myself that I was comfortable with. This didn't mean that I was able to keep the two worlds completely separate. Apparently, there were some people, even journalists, booking in to A&E to try to see me, wasting hospital time in the hope of getting a scoop. To avoid becoming a distraction for my colleagues, I was often placed in the 'resus' unit, which is where the most unwell patients are cared for. I just wanted to get on with my job, but I felt a sense of distance from myself and from the work that I wanted to do. Something told me that I should take a break from medicine in order to come to terms with the changes in my life and understand where my decisions had taken me.

This left me even more shaken than when I first left the show. At least then I'd had the belief that I could return to A&E, but now that my identity as a doctor was slipping away, everything seemed to spiral out of control. I began to feel more and more paranoid because everywhere I turned, I saw people staring or snapping pictures. I started to lose contact with my friends because my frenzied life only ever ruined their nights out. If we met up for a few drinks, it would be no time before the first person would approach our table for a picture and soon groups of drunk people would be circling us. I would do my best to keep them satisfied but I didn't want my friends to spend their evenings working as my minders. So I decided it was best for them if I didn't join. I started to spend my evenings alone, watching other people's lives from across a social media divide as they enjoyed themselves. I became something of a recluse.

I don't believe social media offers an effective antidote to loneliness even though as a culture, we have normalised it. It can be a useful source of information, and I have built a career on the opportunities it offers in this area, but if you are sad from a lack of genuine human connection, seeing your friends' online lives does little to remedy it. Technology can make us feel as if we are connected to those we care about but for me, it felt like a hollow projection of social life. I felt like I was living in a glass box, separated from my friends in the real world. Social media simply offered a new pane of glass through which I could watch them.

It was only once I began to treat social media as a tool for external communication that I started to experience a healthier relationship with it. I decided to see it as an outlet for my professional ambitions as a medical communicator rather than a substitute for my social life, and this at least offset some of the sadness I felt at the challenges I was experiencing in my medical career. So I began to post about healthcare and positive mental health practices. In many ways, I was going on my own mental health journey and I communicated to others what I had learned for myself. I found a team who could help me create informative content and I allowed myself to enjoy their company and the sense of usefulness that I had thought I had lost, but it was still some time before I grew comfortable with my new social and professional life.

There is a certain loneliness to being a content creator. If you are a perfectionist, as I am, and prone to attaching your internal sense of self-worth to external validation, as I often have, it can be a stressful path to choose. In most jobs, there is a certain degree of nuance when it comes to monitoring your performance: you know if you are working hard and other people around you work with you to achieve your collective goals. This is not the case as a social media creator because every piece of work you do has a numerical value that classifies it as successful or not, as good or bad content. On top of that, the work that you create is attached to your identity because you have presented a version of yourself to the world, to be appreciated or ignored by those who encounter it. If you see the success of your content as a reflection of your personality or self-worth, your foundations become insecure. In any walk of life, we must try to have a stable sense of ourselves, to avoid developing a higher sense of ourselves when our work goes well or a lower one when it does not. We must attempt to keep a consistent internal locus of evaluation. In any public-facing work, and particularly as an online creator, this is very important.

I have only learned to manage this over time. The metrics that matter to me now are not really metrics at all – what matters are the conversations I have with people, who let me know which aspects of my work are useful and what they would like me to discuss on my channels. This is still an external form of evaluation, but it is closer to the normal forms of social validation that our minds are built for. It is healthy to feel glad when we make other people feel happy or better informed, but our dopamine systems and a sense of self are not built to derive meaning from clicks. This aspect of social media provides a shallow form of feedback that leaves us with a more shallow sense of our work and worth than we can gain from human interactions.

The truth is that improving my relationship with social media and finding a degree of balance and satisfaction in the work I do there could not override the sense of isolation I felt in the real world. Last year was one of the loneliest years of my life, and although my career as a mental fitness ambassador was going well, my personal life was not. I had never really come to terms with my post-*Love Island* existence and had simply put those problems to one side to focus on the challenges of the pandemic and the grief I experienced when I lost my brother. I had been lonely throughout those times, but I had probably been too busy or too focused on staying afloat to realise it. When the years of the pandemic were over and I had come to an acceptance of my grief, I was left with a realisation that my social world had grown incredibly small. At first, I thought it strange that I only became aware of my loneliness *after* a global pandemic and the grief of losing my brother, but with time, it made sense to me. Working in A&E through the pandemic felt like working in a war zone. I spent a year in almost total isolation outside of my work and team, and for some time afterwards, I was too busy processing my grief and sense of loss to think about the less noticeable losses in my social world. When the threat of the pandemic receded and the shroud of grief lifted, I realised that for all I had fought through those hard times, I had lost the simple joys of friendship.

Some of this was also due to life changes that many of us have to navigate as we move out of our twenties, but the pandemic had both frozen and accelerated my perception of time. I had entered it as a twenty-nine-year-old who liked to meet people for drinks and left it as a thirty-year-old whose friends were now settled with children and had moved to the countryside. I'd always had a small, intimate group of friends but it had grown smaller since the pandemic, as I had pushed away those who remained. In truth, I was struggling mentally and I withdrew. I struggled, and still struggle, to work out how to restart my social life. Whereas at one time, I could give myself a (false) sense of community by drinking with people, once I became sober, I lacked that purpose or access to the ways in which alcohol limited my social anxiety.

I cannot only blame my isolation on my social anxiety, sobriety or the passage of time; I have to take some responsibility for the fact that I have not prioritised my social relationships in the years since the pandemic. It dawned on me one day last year as I walked around Battersea Park that I had a hundred thousand people who might respond to an Instagram post, but not one person to meet with in the park. Where some people might look at the world I had built on social media and think I had so much, I looked out at that park and felt like I had so little. I saw that I was desperately lonely.

I had sacrificed the relationships I had for social media connections. As I have mentioned before, this is not a direct substitute but it is a strangely difficult one to disentangle. The work I do online is deeply personal, it is more honest and intimate than I often am with people I have known for years, and as a result, I expend some of my social energy on that work. People who follow me get to know me in a way that usually only friends do, but I don't draw the wellbeing benefits of social connection from my online life. I am like a friend to millions and I love that fact, but I don't derive the benefits of friendship from this – more a sort of hyper-personal professional satisfaction.

The truth is that I have fewer clear solutions to the challenges I describe in this chapter than any other in the book. It is the one aspect of my life that is most clearly a work in progress, and it is the one in which I feel most detached from what is normal. The only reason I have a platform to talk about my experiences is because I work very hard, and the reality of working hard is that you will have far less time and energy at the end of each day to spend quality time with people you care about. If you are an introvert, as I am, and you recharge by spending time on your own, this is particularly pronounced. If your work also utilises a degree of social energy but keeps you from making new friends, then, well, you see how I feel stuck sometimes.

I have to prioritise finding time in my life for old friends and for making new ones. Sometimes, this may come at the expense of the work I do and I have to accept that. No one can have it all. So I am committing to my friendships because I have grown tired of being lonely. My work, which makes me incredibly proud, is not enough on its own to make me fulfilled. I have to be active in creating genuine connections. I think this is true for most healthy things in our lives because in the modern world there are so many forces that will leave us unhealthy and unhappy if we are passive.

In the case of social connection, I think it is important to understand exactly why and how much we *need* it. In my grandmother's generation in Wales, a community was necessary for survival. They were farmers and at various points in the year, there could be thirty people on each other's farms, doing the same work to make sure the harvest came in or the seeds were sown. The community was essential. Many of us in today's world don't need our community for survival but it's still crucial for our wellbeing. Although we may not need others to survive, we need them to really *live*.

So many of the transitions toward convenience in our society come at the expense of community and social connectedness, and I will admit to not having really thought it through until now. Whereas not long ago, it might have been normal to walk to a shop and engage in conversation with a shopkeeper to get a carton of milk or a newspaper, now I can have my groceries delivered to me with a click of a button or access the news by opening up an app on my phone. This convenience comes at a cost: you've lost the social connection at the shop, the health benefits of the steps and the time spent outside on the walk.

So I'm trying to take the view that these easy options, these new norms that prioritise immediacy over connection, are not always the best routes towards a more meaningful life. In the same way that dopamine-inducing foods are easily accessible but unsatisfying in the long term, so too is a convenient interpersonal life. It takes effort to cultivate a sense of community, in the same way that it takes effort to cultivate a healthy body through exercise, and it is no less important in terms of my mental and physical health. In multiple studies, loneliness and social isolation have been shown to reduce life expectancy, and I find it helps me in some ways to understand it as a health issue. Researchers estimate that social isolation has the same impact on health outcomes as smoking fifteen cigarettes a day, so I have to go cold turkey on my habit of withdrawing.

I find it difficult to cultivate new senses of community because I live in a big city and my working life is quite an isolated one. But that's no reason not to seek out meaningful connections – if anything, it makes the effort more important. This is not just an emotional or social issue, it is a question of health for mind and body.

I have found that making connections through my hobbies has worked for me. I love running, so I now try to join community running groups like the Scrambled Legs or the Friday Night Lights. They create social events built around running and offer a great way for me to meet like-minded people. The latter is particularly good for me, as they are focused on offering a 'night out' vibe, which as an ex-drinker, I often miss. While I could still go to a pub on a Friday night, I feel less of a sense of community when everyone else ends up getting quite drunk while I remain sober. I'm sure lots of ex-drinkers feel differently, but for me, it is not that fun. The benefit of a running club night out is that you still experience the hedonism and the altered states of consciousness that people usually access through alcohol, but replaced by endorphins.

When I attended Friday Night Lights for the first time, I felt the same anxiety weighing on me as I did in the lead up to rugby practice as a teenager. I didn't have a supportive friend to pull me through, but I was able to play that role for myself and managed to counsel the more anxious parts of my mind. I'm beginning to realise that new situations will always present some discomfort for me, and that I have to see that as a challenge I have to overcome for my happiness and my health. Just like we may have to push ourselves to go to the gym or for a run, we have to take ownership of our mind and motivation when approaching social situations we know are good for us. I also find it helps to choose activities where I can access the dopamine that has so often been a driver of unhealthy habits for me.

Running is one of my dopamine drivers and riding motorbikes is another. I have started to join social situations that are based on a love of riding motorbikes because the high I enjoy from that activity helps to counteract the social anxiety I feel around joining in. Bike-lovers are a community where shared interests and dopamine highs bond people very deeply, and this is my blueprint for building social connections in a modern world that can be isolating. As a culture, and particularly in increasingly atomised cities, we need to be conscious of the groups and activities that can counteract the public health issue of isolation, but it is up to us as individuals to join in. If you can, go further and create the community you would like to see in the world.

Joining in is what I intend to do, as well as being active in maintaining the older friendships that I have often neglected. Discussing this subject has made it clear to me that there are steps I need to take to improve this aspect of my life. Instead of complaining about my friends moving out of London, I need to make the effort to travel to see them. Instead of feeling envy when I see people with bigger friendships groups enjoying themselves on social media, I need to turn that energy into a more productive emotion because if it doesn't motivate me to be a better and more diligent friend then my time and energy have been wasted. Finally, I have to accept that my work–life balance needs to be redressed and that friendship needs to be a priority. This can be hard for me to accept, and in our culture it's a slightly taboo thing to say, but our friendships are more important than our jobs. This should be the norm. If prioritising my connections means posting less or committing to fewer speaking engagements, then so be it. I have worked at the expense of my social connections for too long and I have realised that my work alone cannot make me happy, so I have to recalibrate the balance.

My loneliness stems from a sense of powerlessness, and from the very normal reaction to the difference between how my social life is and what I expect it to be. I see now that the only antidotes to that powerlessness are self-knowledge, bravery and the application of those two things in the pursuit of community. The knowledge of how and why I hold myself back from a better, more connected life and the bravery to take the steps I know will help me lead me to one. If you feel similarly to me, I encourage you to try as I am trying now. Make an effort to spend time with those who care about you and normalise experiences where you meet like-minded people who you will grow to care about in time. Do things you love and meet new people in the process.

There is nothing to lose and everything to gain.

7

HOW WAS THE PANDEMIC FOR YOU?

Life has a tendency to take us off script. There is no amount of foresight that can prepare us entirely for the events that change our course and no amount of planning that would make navigating them forever painless. At times like this, my tendency to operate in the moment rather than carefully plan ahead can come in handy. When the Covid pandemic hit, it certainly felt like that was the case. No amount of planning could have prepared us for a reality we couldn't understand; no amount of imagination could have given us a sense of what was to come.

I adjusted to the necessities of the pandemic in the way that I always do – by throwing myself into it head first and without much thought. This was a scenario, like A&E medicine, where I felt comfortable in chaos. We were all frightened and uncomfortable due to the lack of understanding we had about the social, emotional and medical situation we were in, but I found a simplified sense of purpose. I only had one thing to do and that was to offer my services in A&E. I had a sense of duty and in many ways I was grateful for that.

I think that being a frontline worker made adjusting to the pandemic more straightforward for me in certain ways – the 'new normal' was like a supercharged version of my old one. Controlling the controllables came to the fore and I was able to focus on what I could do rather than on what was lost. For my friends and family, there was the fear of what the pandemic could do but also a sense of their own powerlessness. People like to feel useful, we like to have purpose, so to be told that there is something dangerous happening at a global scale and that the most you can do is sit at home creates a great deal of nervous tension. People simply watched the news and hoped, which felt like the closest thing to making a contribution when everyone was being asked to do as little as possible.

When we feel threatened, we often only feel better by taking action. For example, if I am anxious, I find that the best thing I can do to calm my mind is walk, because moving my body creates balance in my racing mind. This is why it is easier to think through problems when we take a walk, as walking feels like a response to the threat we perceive or the opportunities our mind is telling us we might miss. During the pandemic, people were told they faced a threat and were asked to stay still, which feels counterintuitive and only added a sense of claustrophobia to the anxiety they experienced. I felt fortunate that even though I faced the same fears as the rest of the country, I could find the sense of purpose that comes with taking action. I may have been travelling to the very place that everyone else wanted to avoid, putting myself in proximity to the virus in a time of social distancing, but I knew the hospital was the best place I could be. I was grateful that given the choice between confronting danger or trying to keep it at arm's length, I was able to choose the path of action.

Still, it was a challenging time to be a medic. We were operating at the edge of our understanding and our capacity, so we had to learn on the job in the most highly pressurised circumstances. In the beginning, for example, we were very careful to protect and segregate asthma patients, as everything we knew about respiratory systems told us that they would be particularly vulnerable to the virus. It was a shock to us when the data started to come in showing that asthmatics who were medicated with steroids were outperforming all of our expectations, and we had to shift our priorities and resources to other, more vulnerable groups.

We wanted to be careful not to give patients too much fluid in those early days but soon we realised how important it was to protect people's kidneys through hydration, so again we changed tack. We were operating at the frontline in the physical sense of being people's first recourse when they became seriously ill, but also in terms of time. We met society's problems first and discovered new information about the virus before others did. This meant that we saw the spikes in infections when they were still only just small upticks and foresaw the capacity issues when they were just increasing patient numbers. Other people's fears were our reality, but I felt lucky because reality is easier to act on than fear.

I decided to try to mediate between the reality of our frontline and the fear that people were experiencing in the isolation of their homes. I wanted to communicate what doctors were doing and what we needed, so I agreed to start doing interviews with media organisations during work breaks and at lunchtime. This was a very strange experience but I didn't have the time or resources to dwell on its novelty.

Once, I was on *BBC News at Ten* but still in my scrubs taking care of patients at 21:55. I had to leave the resus unit and change in the family waiting room, where I would conduct the interview. It was surreal, stepping out of one role where I was trying to save someone's life and into another where I was sending a dispatch to millions of frightened people. I can still feel the producers panicking around me, sense the nervous energy at that time and remember well the unspoken understanding that somehow the news, like doctors, was more important than it had ever been. It felt strange that something so grand and serious could be as simple as taking a video call in a waiting room. Looking back, it probably wasn't the most polished news segment but I was comfortable with that because my profession was in the next room. I had more important things to do. The producers found it strange that I was not in thrall to the seriousness of being on the news, but in my mind it was simple. There was nothing as serious as what was going on in the ward next door and if that meant I seemed strangely relaxed about being on the news, I was comfortable with it. All I could do was answer their questions. Those questions mostly amounted to: *What is this sickness? Will we be all right? When?* And the truth was that I could only respond to the best of my ability.

We knew even then that it would be months and years before we could really describe the impacts of the virus, understand immunity and grasp how long it would take us to recover as a society. I could only provide a voice from the other side, like a war reporter or some astronaut beaming down from a shuttle, to let the world know that we were here, doing our best, and that we intended to continue doing so. I couldn't really tell them what they wanted to know, which was how our society would cope.

In fact, I think we're still trying to understand the impact of the pandemic on a societal and individual level. Although we know more about the individual health impacts of the virus, we are still working to appreciate all the changes it wrought in our lives – on children's education, on our ways of working, on our economies and our minds. Of all those impacts, it is the way the pandemic affected our minds that I have thought about most (given my work in mental health since), and here I find it useful to think about the role of dopamine.

Dopamine has been described as the neurochemical that deals with *wanting* rather than *having*. It's also why we may feel intense craving (wanting) for something such as alcohol or a coveted new item of clothing but feel curiously flat when we get it. It's also why our desire for something addictive can continue even when our brain no longer gets the same level of reward from it.

The interesting thing about the pandemic and dopamine is that we were put in a constant state of wanting things that we couldn't have. Whereas the difficult dopamine relationships I have described revolve around wanting easily accessible but often harmful things, the pandemic was characterised by an unsatisfied desire for good, healthy things. We wanted to socialise, dance, play sports or hug our friends and extended family, so we had an active but unresolved relationship with dopamine. While this constitutes a very normal sense of longing in truly abnormal circumstances and is the opposite of addiction, many people did turn to less healthy dopamine-driven behaviours in the pandemic, and I think it could be argued that this was in part because we had less access to the healthy, sociable things we wanted.

Many people have cited the growth of online shopping and compulsive buying in the pandemic as an example of how we substituted an unhealthy practice for the healthy ones we could not experience. For a lot of us, online shopping became an outlet. I'm not trying to demonise people buying things on the internet. Purchasing things online can be incredibly useful and we really only need to consider it a problem if it is out of control, leads to a decreased sense of wellbeing and negatively impacts someone's life.

There are many reasons why people develop compulsive habits, but for shopping addictions experts often cite boredom, loneliness, depression and anxiety as key factors. The pandemic presented a new form of boredom, as well as a whole new kind of anxiety. This created the perfect psychological conditions for people to seek dopamine rewards from shopping, facilitated by all the new online market-places that offered greater opportunities for the habit to develop.

I am clearly in no position to demonise social media but I also believe the pandemic led many people to develop unhealthy relationships with digital platforms. There is an even clearer link between social media addiction and the isolation of the pandemic than other forms of compulsive behaviour, as it's almost a direct substitute for the human connection that people lost. As someone who has been lonely and disconnected, and who continues to manage my relationship with social media, it is a subject close to my heart.

The pandemic created a huge surge in social media usage. For many of us, these platforms were a window to the world, a connection to all of the living rooms and kitchens in which the rest of human life seemed to be taking place. This was not necessarily a bad thing: it could be a mindful practice, something that we chose to do for entertainment and some semblance of connection. It only becomes an addiction when it is an urge rather than a choice. While many people may have decided to use social media more in the pandemic, the reward system that it created was a powerful one because we were finding so few rewards elsewhere. This meant that even when normal life resumed and our more traditionally rewarding behaviours, like socialising and enjoying the outdoors, became available to us again, many people found them less attractive relative to the dopamine hit of using social media. We strengthened our attachment to it and in doing so may have weakened our attachment to other things.

This was certainly the case for me. While I continued to work at the hospital throughout the pandemic, I still experienced the sense of isolation that many other people did. Work did not feel like a place for socialising. In normal circumstances, I might find time to stop and speak with my colleagues or to spend time with them when their shifts finish, but during the Covid response, we were so stretched that none of this was possible. I also didn't really get to connect with patients in the manner I was used to. Doctors and patients often develop relationships close to friendship, forged over weeks or months of contact and conversation, but during the pandemic, the demands on our time were such that there was no way to stop and get to know the people we were caring for. So while I was lucky to leave the house and have a job that provided me with purpose, it was not the same job that I had once known, and it offered little of the personal or social connection that otherwise makes it feel so worthwhile.

Outside of my work hours, I was more isolated than ever and social media became my only link to the wider world. I would finish my shift and cycle back to my flat, where I knew I would be alone until the next shift began. At home, I would eat a quick meal and settle down to work on my social media videos. This meant thinking about the subjects I would cover in the videos over the next week, recording those that would be released in a few days and editing those I had already recorded to release that evening. From 6pm until around midnight, I would be in a small, dark room, but my mind would be racing and my thoughts would travel to all corners of the world. Social media was fast becoming my job and my link to all the people that I might otherwise have spoken to if circumstances were different. I did develop some unhealthy attachments to it but they were not as significant as dependencies I have created at other times and in other areas of my life. For example, in those early days, I definitely let my mood and self-image rise and fall with the numbers on the screen. I felt anticipation and excitement at the release of a new video (dopamine) and an incredible rush when people responded. I grew disappointed if they did not. This was imperfect and I now see these aspects as part of my path to becoming a creator, and something that I could manage through a degree of mindfulness.

I was old enough, and my brain was developed enough, for me to manage the connections between self-image and social media use. But I think this relationship is most challenging for young people, who, in a critical stage of their brain development, struggle to separate their fragile sense of self from the tens, hundreds or thousands of responses they receive. All of the data I've seen suggests that social media can be very harmful to teenagers, so I would argue that decisive measures should be taken to protect their developing minds. We should normalise the teaching of digital literacy, which is an educational challenge that we have not quite adapted to, given that technology develops faster than school curricula.

Social media companies should also be required to provide a more age-appropriate experience for young users, which limits the amount of feedback children receive, as well as more effective mechanisms to stop younger people getting around age restrictions. I would recommend that parental oversight is built into app usage. I also hope parents can feel empowered to keep their children away from social media if they think it is not in their best interests, and that we can find a way to reduce the social pressures on children to be consumers and creators in this digital economy. I believe that social media is an avenue for many young people to exercise their innate drive towards creativity rather than simply an expression of vanity. To this end, greater access to creative pursuits like music, dance and art for teenagers would actually do as much to help children develop a healthy relationship with social media as limiting their use of it would. As this is not my area of expertise, I recommend the work of people like Jonathan Haidt or Lucy Foulkes if you would like to read a deeper discussion of the challenges that young people face today.

We can often fill holes in our experience with compulsive behaviours. Pain or loneliness provide fertile ground for compulsive behaviours to take hold because they offer small, manageable rewards in an existence that does not feel broadly rewarding. I think my loneliness during the pandemic manifested as an over-reliance on social media, but not for social media's sake. I think it was actually a conduit for the work addiction that I have struggled with my whole life. I have often turned to work as an antidote to my poor self-image, and the loneliness and unhappiness that comes with it. For me, the cycle is clear, though for all that it is evidently an unsuccessful route to life satisfaction, I remain within it. The cycle goes like this:

1. I have experienced low self-esteem since childhood.
2. So I work hard to experience success that will convince me that I am in fact worthwhile.
3. I work so hard that I eventually burn myself out.
4. When I am burned out, I grow unhappy and become self-critical.
5. I experience low self-esteem and . . . the cycle begins again.

In light of this cycle, it's clear that social media was not necessarily my problem but the vehicle through which I acted out an unhealthy pattern of behaviour. The underlying issue of my low self-esteem can interact with any number of harmful behaviours – and it has, from alcohol misuse to forms of disordered eating. It's simply that my work addiction has been the most consistent response to it. While things like drug misuse or gambling addiction are clearly harmful, and rarely generate positive outcomes that others can appreciate, my addiction to work (and to a lesser extent social media) has been both a compulsive response to my mental health challenges *and* the basis of the success I have had and the esteem I receive. I have a problem that is inextricably linked to the good things I do, which does present some other issues in trying to untangle it.

It's clear to me that I enjoy the positive impacts I can have in the world but, somehow, I have to separate those from the unhappiness that created the conditions for my drive and relentless working habits. I have to believe that I can be both happy and driven, even if my drive has always stemmed from a misplaced belief that I need to work myself into a place of self-respect. My achievements will never be enough to give me lasting happiness – which I think is true for most of us. So I think I need to appreciate myself first and find a drive that is built on more positive foundations. I'm certainly working towards that now but it is a continuing process, and just as I had to be conscious of it as a medical student, doctor and burgeoning social media creator, I have to be conscious of it now.

The most obvious way that we can reset our dopamine response

and reduce our compulsive behaviours is through abstinence.* In
some ways, it seems counterintuitive because we think denying
ourselves the things we want only makes us want them more, but
that is only a short-term effect. In the long term, if we can break the
cycle of feeding our desire (the dopamine response), then our brains
can develop a more balanced relationship to the object of it.

This is where another resource in impulse control comes
in: mindfulness. This is the practice of observing our minds
impassively and without judgement. When we neutrally consider
our responses in the context of dopamine-driven behaviours (like
mindless scrolling or impulse buying), we often see that we've been
acting on an unconscious level, compulsively or impulsively, and
that we don't actually feel rewarded. If we introduce mindfulness,
we can take back a degree of control over our impulses. This then
resets our dopamine system and allows us to more mindfully enjoy
things that we crave less but get more from. People often think
mindfulness is an esoteric practice that involves staring at rivers or
hugging trees, but in fact it is more that observing our minds and
our responses opens up space to enjoy such things. No one craves a
river but everyone can enjoy one.

What I find interesting is that mindfulness often gets equated
to meditating. Of course, meditation is a form of mindfulness but
there are so many different ways to apply mindfulness in our daily
lives. The end goal as I understand it is to be present. In the moment.

---

*   Although, not in all cases – for example, substance misuse disorders
     require the clinical advice and oversight of an expert to help manage
     withdrawal.

Our bodies and its organs only ever exist in the present, which is why breathwork is so helpful, as by tuning into our breathing we are becoming present, because our lungs are not in the past or future! How we become present varies from person to person. Mindfulness is sitting reading, its riding a motorbike (one of my faves), stomping in the park listening to the birds, looking at the trees, feeling the wind in my face. Anything that brings us to 'the Now' (as Eckhart Tolle would say). I find a cold shower is a great instant way to come to the present. For some people, it could be playing an instrument. What I want people to understand is the importance of the goal, rather than the method.

Almost all suffering is the result of worrying about the future or ruminating about the past. How often is your problem something that you are facing in the Now? The sad reality is that most of us spend our lives suffering as a result of things that are not happening in the moment we are actually in. People can lose their huge chunks of their lives to worry, for example. I have lost years! As Owen Kane describes in his book *Addicted to Anxiety*, we are quite literally hooked on it. No one chooses to wake up anxious – why would anyone want that? But our brains become wired and programmed to worry, as if worrying will protect us. Mindfulness is about breaking that loop, returning us to the now so we can live our lives. Ideally, we should aim for one big activity in our day – such as a good walk, run, playing the piano or whatever we find helpful – and multiple small resets – such as breathwork or grounding exercises – to calm our minds and break the worry cycle. As an ADHDer, for me, it's about picking the tool that I can stick too, which is why I generally choose movement or activity-based things.

I hope that this practice of learning to watch our minds with a certain amount of distance becomes normal, and I have tried to advocate for children learning mindfulness as their brains are developing. Mindful awareness of our dopamine-driven behaviours really is a better route to improved mental health.

When it comes to my own mental health, and the habits that feed in or take away from it, I find it helps to think both in terms of long-term and short-term practices. The way that I have just described my relationship to work is an example of a long-term view that generates understanding because I am looking at factors from my childhood that inform that pattern of behaviour and trying to create new approaches that will improve my future. This helps me to understand why I engage in compulsive habits, but it is focusing on short-term behaviours that helps me know how to break compulsions.

Most of us have some compulsive behaviours. You might check your phone every five minutes for messages or scroll through the same news website multiple times a day. Maybe you find yourself buying and returning far more things than you would ever need or you struggle to pass a cafe without buying yourself a treat. None of these things are bad in and of themselves, but it's always helpful to be conscious of our behaviours, so that they remain a choice rather than a compulsion.

This is particularly relevant in the twenty-first century because our brains are constantly stimulated by technology and marketing that is designed to create a dopamine response. The modern world is geared to make us want things, to gamble, drink, scroll or buy coffees, and it is only by being conscious of how our brains respond to stimuli that we can have balance and a degree of ownership over our own minds.

Psychotherapists talk about breaking the stimulus–response cycle. To do this, we need to practise self-reflection to increase the scope of our actions beyond a purely responsive existence. When our existence is dominated by responses to stimuli (and particularly dopamine, or wanting), we have very little room to do anything much other than fulfil these constant, small urges, making it harder to see the bigger picture. To enjoy a life that feels meaningful, we must step outside the stimulus–response cycle to give ourselves the time and space we need to decide on what a meaningful life is to us. Many of us feel like we do not have time to stop and think, but that is at least in part because we spent so much time moving unthinkingly in the service of our dopamine system.

This is something that we all need to actively manage and be willing to work at. Our dopamine responses are controlled by something called our limbic system, which is a very powerful driver of motivation and behaviour. To gain the control of our limbic system that is necessary to allow ourselves space to pause and reflect on our happiness (or otherwise) would be a significant challenge even if that very system were not being manipulated every day and from every direction. This manipulation has been described as 'limbic capitalism' by author David Courtwright. In our world, control of our dopamine responses is the main driver of most consumer businesses. Limbic capitalism includes advertising or marketing, but it is much more than that: it incorporates everything from the way our technology is designed to keep us scrolling to the way our food is mass produced to keep us hungry. It is a culture built upon wanting and it leaves us wanting, in both senses of the word. The simple fact is that if we live without stopping to examine our minds, we live at its mercy, thrown between the dopamine spikes of stimulus (advertisement/social media notification) and action (alcohol/fast food/endless scrolling), and at some point, our mind is no longer our own. I know this sounds very heavy but I would argue that one of the most certain routes to empowerment, self-ownership and health is through an awareness of our limbic system and dopamine responses, and learning to adopt approaches that allow us to make decisions that are not driven by external stimuli.

The normalisation of limbic capitalism has been a steady process in the last hundred years and we need a concerted public effort if we are to change our society to develop new norms which free us from this manipulation. The good news is that there are precedents: for example, cigarette smoking used to be perfectly normal but we've moved to a much healthier norm where it's now considered a harmful addiction. It took time to define cigarettes as something harmful and addictive before this norm could be changed. Fortunately, the language of addiction is already prevalent in discussions of things like gambling, shopping and substance abuse, but it may help to introduce it more routinely to other types of consumption.

The next step in denormalising our limbic capitalist system, our culture of addiction that touches almost every aspect of our lives, is to campaign for restrictions on marketing. If we think about how tobacco packaging has been changed to make cigarettes less appealing, this could offer a blueprint for how processed food or other consumer products are marketed. Selling products and lifestyles through bright colours and aspirational images is something we have to reconsider in our society, particularly if what is being sold can be harmful or addictive. Any restrictions we place on dopamine-driven marketing should be particularly focused on advertising aimed at children, as their developing brains are particularly susceptible to manipulation.

Finally, and importantly – because we need positive solutions to these issues – access to positive, non-addicting goods should be encouraged. While we decrease the opportunities for effective marketing of harmful products, we should offer opportunities and subsidies for those marketing healthy and empowering habits, hobbies or goods. Healthy foods should be free to stand out in the supermarket, just as fruits and vegetables naturally would in the wild. Books and magazines, exercise equipment and pro-social games and toys could be marketed in fun, lively ways that spike dopamine and allow them to compete with less healthy products that are sold to us through dopamine manipulation. Taxing unhealthy products could raise funds to support group activities like sports, drama and music, which help people to build a sense of community, learn skills and become more physically and mentally healthy.

Decades of unchecked limbic capitalism has seen many of us fall into patterns of dependency, isolation and disconnection, so our aim should be to encourage ways of eating, socialising and relaxing that bring people together and offer individuals benefits, rather than maximise profits for those who manipulate them.

Of course, we also have to be conscious of what we can do as individuals to create a society in which it is normal to be free from the forms of addiction that we have normalised. As a person with a neurodevelopmental condition that involves a dysregulated limbic system, I have struggled with creating this new normal, but in the process of figuring out what works for me I have learned that there are behavioural, psychological and physical actions we can take to reclaim our attention and compulsion. We have discussed how abstinence and mindfulness are the most powerful regulators of your dopamine response. If you find yourself mindlessly scrolling, for example, be aware of it and accept that you may be better off putting your phone in another room for a certain amount of time each day. Very quickly, your brain will reorient to no longer expect the regular dopamine hit of a WhatsApp notification or news updates and you'll find yourself wanting them less and scrolling less.

Try to exercise, in a way that suits you. Exercise regulates and increases your dopamine receptors, so that if they have become overused and overrun by the constant stimulation in our world you can create space to have new dopamine responses to different things – things that you actually *want* to want. Meditation or mindfulness practice is also very powerful because, like exercise, it raises our dopamine levels through self-directed practice, which helps us wrest back control of our limbic system from advertising and technology.

I would also recommend trying to do difficult things for the sake of their difficulty. This sounds counterintuitive, but by learning to enjoy doing things that are harder to master we will change our reward systems. We often find that unhealthy, dopamine-driven behaviours become unrewarding after a time, but by using our dopamine system for its true purpose, to drive us towards good and difficult things, we can recalibrate it.

There are some convincing arguments about how we can develop a more balanced and regulated dopamine system. The psychiatrist Anna Lembke, author of *Dopamine Nation,* is very clear that we should be far more careful about our smartphone usage than what is considered normal now. She describes the smartphone as a sort of 'hypodermic needle' of 'dopamine delivery' that creates both dependency and leaves us in a dopamine-deficient state. This is deeply problematic as we need our dopamine system for motivation to do all manner of difficult, satisfying and healthy tasks, and if we are constantly overloading it with notifications then the system grows depleted.

We should also be conscious of our circadian rhythms, which are the mechanism by which our bodies regulate the timing of physical functions – the most obvious of which are waking and sleeping. Dopamine spikes have the potential to dysregulate these rhythms so we should be careful not to spike our dopamine close to sleeping. This can become a sort of vicious cycle, as poor sleep and disrupted circadian rhythms also impact our body's ability to regulate dopamine itself. So when we have a disrupted circadian cycle, we are more likely to engage in impulsive behaviours.

Fortunately, we are able to regulate our circadian rhythms through access to sunlight and darkness. Sunlight impacts many aspects of our neurochemistry: it makes us produce serotonin, lowers cortisol (your stress response) and orders our circadian rhythms (which will help you sleep later). In short, it improves your mood, helps you sleep and gives you greater control over your impulses throughout the day – and when you get outside in the daylight, you also get all the benefits of a walk.

The benefits of morning sunlight to our sleep should not be underestimated, as the time that we fall asleep and how we sleep have a big impact on our wellbeing and dopamine systems. We should also be aware of how we behave later in the day for this reason. We should try to avoid technology and bright lights in the evening, and always after 10pm. If we can create consistent circadian rhythms (the patterns of wakefulness and sleepiness), we will be healthier in a number of measures, but particularly in terms of our compulsions and cravings.

These are components of living healthily, rather than avoiding sickness. If there is any norm that I have sought to question in my professional and personal life, it is the view that there are two states of being, healthy and sick, and any measure to promote the former is only to stave off the latter. I would argue that there is a whole world of experience that exists in between sickness and health, and that the more that we focus on what it is to live well, happily and healthily, the better we will all be. We should not only exercise to avoid injury (although it is incredibly good for that), we should also do it because it is enjoyable, it makes us healthier and it opens up our range of possibilities. We should not eat vegetables to avoid getting diabetes, but because they provide us with the nutrition that allows us to live a happier, active and energetic life. Pursuing health is much more enjoyable than avoiding sickness.

Health is freedom and we have the freedom to grow healthier, whatever our life circumstances. The problem with the binary that separates sickness and health is that it offers very little room for gradual progression, the joy of a journey in which we see that we are more capable than we were yesterday – healthier and able to do more through self-love and effort.

For most of us, this is within our control. We can take steps to grow healthier, feel proud of ourselves and show that we value our minds and bodies enough to make an effort on our own behalf. I am not recommending that we all do Ironmans or climb Everest, but to try to live a little healthier every day. Maybe that means a few more steps or a few more greens, but it is an investment we can make in ourselves because we think we deserve it. The key is not looking at healthy practices as subtractions (no more fast food/ no more Netflix nights) but *additions*. The opportunity to enjoy that fast food when we have it, safe in the knowledge that we have respected our mind and body, or the ability to enjoy that moment on the sofa in a body that feels the warm buzz of endorphins.

We don't need to take away our smartphones; we need to find something more enjoyable and healthier to do with our time. Often, this means looking at ourselves and what truly makes us happy. Going for a walk instead of scrolling when we wake up may seem less tempting, but once we have tried it a few times we are almost guaranteed to realise it makes us feel happier and healthier. Instead of thinking that we are removing our rewards (by changing our dopamine systems), we can think about how much more rewarding it feels when we do something that requires self-motivation.

There is nothing more enjoyable than getting better at something, but if we give our minds and bodies up to entertainment, tech or fast-food companies, we will not have the energy to experience that progress. So see if you can make progress itself tempting, because the cycle of effort and reward tends to become compulsive in its own right. It is certainly more satisfying and undoubtedly healthier. These may seem like grand ideas but really they boil down to small practices that bring our happiness back into our own control.

This means that although life has a tendency to take us off script, we can still be the authors of our own existence. Events may be outside of our control, but the small actions that make up a lifetime still remain within it. We have to choose whether we want to spend our lives responding to stimuli or creating our own meaning. I know which one I prefer. Even though it may seem hard at first, it will be infinitely more satisfying because our dissatisfaction stems from the easy things.

I hope that some of my advice helps you on this journey that I am also taking, to have ownership over my own mind. The pandemic taught me a lot about how we value freedom and control over our lives – now we have a chance to put that knowledge into action.

8

ARE YOU GRIEVING?

People assume that the most difficult thing about being a key worker in the pandemic was where we had to be, when in fact it was where we couldn't be that caused the most pain for me. I could not be with my brother in the last year of his life and it was only when he died that I realised how much I, and many others, had sacrificed. I made the choice to work and isolate myself throughout the pandemic. I couldn't travel to Wales to be with my family, so my year was split between the clamour of an A&E ward and the silence of an empty flat. I wanted to be useful at that difficult time but I only realised later that it came at the expense of being with the people I loved.

The last time I saw my brother Llŷr was a few weeks before the first lockdown. He was preparing to embark on his own medical studies and so had come to shadow me at Lewisham hospital. Before he left, I hugged him at the train station and said goodbye, unaware that it would be the last time we ever saw each other.

Llŷr was similar to me in many ways – sensitive, driven and deeply committed to helping people in need. He spent the year of the pandemic at home, retaking an A-level as I once had, before taking his place at medical school. At the age of nineteen, when he should have had his whole life ahead of him, he took his own life.

There are many aspects of grief and grieving that are strange and defy our expectations. One thing that often strikes me, though, is how the experience can be so disorientating and yet so perfectly memorable; how something that left me numb can feel so rich with jagged detail now that I look back on it. Llŷr died on a sunny July day. We had planned to spend the week together in London but I asked him if we could reschedule because one of my closest friends, Tom, needed support as his father was dying. Llŷr was very understanding and told me that I should be there for Tom. Somehow, in prioritising one death, I missed the signs that another was coming. It's a sad truth that the worst-case scenarios are often beyond our imaginations, and I keep that as a reminder not to dwell on the imaginary because there will be a time when reality requires all of our strength and resolve just to endure.

So I kept my friend Tom company instead of seeing Llŷr in the week before his death. When Tom went home, I made plans to have dinner with some other friends before returning to Wales the next day. The borders had just been reopened and I was excited to see my family for the first time in a year. The dinner with my friends felt normal – strangely normal in hindsight. Looking back, it feels as if it should have been tinged with some recognition that it was the last such experience of my life, the last supper of a youth unmarked by grief. That was not the case, though, and it was perfectly ordinary, until it was not. Halfway through the meal, my father called me and I let it ring through. In my family, we have an understanding that if a person calls once they just want to chat but if they ring twice, it is something serious.

My phone rang again. This time, I answered and asked my father who had died. Somehow, I knew that was the reason he had called but I couldn't prepare for his answer. He told me Llŷr was dead.

It felt as if a grenade had exploded at my feet. It did not kill me but simply stopped time, leaving me neither alive nor dead but struck with a sharp pain, ears ringing, my vision blurred. I had never experienced anything like it. I had always thought that grief would exist in the mind, that it would bear some relation to psychological sadnesses that I had felt previously, but what came now took place on a deeply physical level. It was agony, a bursting through my chest and a dropping in my stomach that continued onwards as if the depths it could plummet to were infinite, as if there was no point at which it could stop.

I left dinner in a daze and went back to my flat. Only then did my father tell me that Llŷr had died by suicide. In a moment, my bodily pain rushed back up to my mind, as the 'what ifs' that I would grow to know so well began to take shape. How had I missed his sadness? Would things be different if I had been there for him that week? Why didn't he tell me that he was in such a difficult place? In our conversations over the preceding weeks, he had told me he felt low, but that was mixed in with more positive thoughts about preparing for university and looking forward to his visit to London. I couldn't reconcile my knowledge of his world with what must have been his reality.

It felt like Llŷr died twice that day: once when my father told me the news and a second time when he explained how it had happened, but the enduring sensation was one of complete and utter shock. My brother Elliott drove to pick me up and we set off together on the five-hour journey back home in complete silence. We played no music and the radio stayed off; we simply stared at the lights on the road and took it in turns to fall into tears. I still hadn't accepted the reality of the situation and I couldn't bring myself to call my parents in fear that it would make it all more real.

The hope that you can somehow defy reality is a cruel trick that grief plays. For many months after Llŷr's death, I hoped that I might be in some long and terrible dream, but there was no keeping reality at bay. I feared going to sleep because upon waking I would have to remember all over again. The truth was worse than any nightmare my subconscious could dream up, and the knowledge deep down that this loss was forever meant that the sadness I felt in the present was tinged with the reminder that this would be my future too. We would carry this loss for a lifetime. His chair at the dinner table would remain forever empty and we would mourn both the present and the futures that we and Llŷr had lost.

I didn't sleep for the first few nights; I lay there with my eyes open in a state of electrified shock. At regular intervals, I was shaken out of it by the terror that it might be true, and then the realisation that it was. After two or three days, exhaustion got the better of me. I felt consumed by a strange sickness that I also saw on the faces of my parents.

In those first few days, a greyness settled upon us, as if Llŷr's death somehow drew from our own lifeforces. Elliott and I quietly discussed our fear that our parents might die of acute grief. They looked like children, wide-eyed and confused by the cruelty of the world, and that was unnerving. I was a grown man but the experience of seeing my parents in a state of such vulnerability added another layer of strangeness to being in my family home. I remember lying in bed and hearing my father hoovering the house in the middle of the night. The sound shot through the pitch-black house like a cry and I simply lay there, listening to it. I knew my dad needed something to do, some small thing that he could control, even if it was only dust on the floor.

I soon realised the responsibility I had to my parents. I needed to be strong, to hide that I was struggling and somehow show that we all had it in us to live our lives again. That sounds like an impossible task but I knew that someone in our house had to retain something like hope. The knowledge of what my parents were experiencing made it clear to me that I needed to support them. While I grieved as a brother, they were parents, makers and nurturers who had lost their youngest son. Just as I loved Llŷr, I loved them, and I knew that their loss was different to mine, so if I could support them, I was doing something in his name. This realisation sparked some of the experience I had as an accident and emergency responder and I knew that I had to at least get them physically through to the funeral. I spoke with my mother about her feelings, but to this day my dad remains silent about what he experienced. In his eyes, there is no amount of light we can shed on the darkness to change it one bit. To him, the only thing we can do is try to move forwards. I will not say that he is wrong, even if my experiences with therapy tell me that talking always helps, that although memories and pain can never be removed, the way we hold them, and they us, can be improved. My father is a product of his time and I cannot claim to understand what he has been through. Llŷr was his best friend. Alongside my mother, he had been the last person to see him and the first to know him. I could not tell him how to grieve.

I would delay my own grieving to help him and my mother endure. I had to be strong enough to help them make it to the funeral, the first milestone in a lifetime of grief that we could at least work towards. So we lived from one hour to the next and focused on planning the funeral. When it came, it was a bleak thing. In July 2020, social distancing protocols were still in place and group gatherings were limited, so there could only be twelve of us, masked and at a distance from one another, mourning the death of a teenager. At a time when we needed community, our group was limited in number and in a moment when we needed closeness above anything else, we were told to keep our distance. It felt like an extra cruelty but one which came as no surprise, given the moment we were in.

Elliott and I spoke at the sparse ceremony. We still didn't really have the words to describe what had happened, as it was happening as we spoke. The life and the loss were only being understood as we walked up to the empty lectern, the grief was being made in front of our eyes, so we were not closing a chapter but writing it. Still, we made it, and sometimes in grief that is all you can ask for. In the context of loss through suicide, that idea takes on extra significance. Continuing to live is not something to be taken lightly – it can be an achievement, particularly in the context of suicide where a person's pain may end but that of their loved ones only grows.

It is not an easy thing to admit but many people who have lost a loved one to suicide will know that anger is a part of your grief. Your thoughts change from one moment to the next, but when someone has taken their own life, there are moments when you think about what they have taken from you and the ones you love. His suicide was a cruel thing, even though it was not his intention to be cruel. My parents had given everything for us; they had worked all their lives and earned the right to enjoy their retirement, but his death took that from them. These things do not make me love him any less, and I don't feel I am doing a disservice to his memory by telling the truth, which is that I have been angry at my younger brother. He suffered deeply but in taking his life, his suffering has been multiplied and passed on. He did not seek to cause pain in taking his life, but it has made for a painful thing. Part of that pain is that anger is now woven into the tapestry of empathy, love and loss that accompanies the death of a loved one.

We do not speak ill of the dead but we must speak truth about the feelings of the living, and I wish that Llŷr could have endured, for his sake and for our family's. I don't like to speculate but I think he believed that the next steps he had to take were simply too much for him. I wish I could have told him to take his time and to lean on us – because what we endured in his loss showed how strong we could be for one another.

After three weeks back at home in Wales, I returned to London. I don't know whether that was the right thing to do but it felt like I couldn't be there any longer. Elliott took on the responsibility of caring for my parents and I know he has carried a heavy burden in the years since. I had been like an emergency responder, first at the scene but willing to pass it on to someone else. An imperfect role but the only one I felt capable of doing. Emergency responders act first and reflect later, and in my grief, this meant burying my feelings until I had helped my family through the immediate shock. It meant acting first and grieving later.

When I arrived back in London, I distracted myself in the only way I knew: by working and drinking. Ninety per cent of my time was spent working – in A&E, on books or on campaigns – and the rest I spent in pubs. I knew I was being avoidant but I was driven by a fear that my grief might break me. Work was numbing but it gave me a part of my identity to hold on to, something outside of my grief that might stop me from falling through the net. I didn't want to be changed or diminished by my grief, I just wanted to be who I was before I got the news, which was another way of saying I wanted Llŷr to be alive.

All of my fears of loss I channelled into a manageable fear that my work was going to fall away, and because that was something I could control, I prioritised it over engaging with my loss. I didn't think I could be happy but believed I could at least retain a sense of purpose through my work. And while I may have been wrong about happiness, I did benefit from keeping my professional life moving forwards. My work in mental health advocacy, in particular, offered me an outlet, a way to talk about positive self-care practice and to feel like I was taking some action in response to my grief. Ideally, I would have worked and also left time outside of work to take stock of how I was feeling, but I don't think the work itself was necessarily a problem. The drinking I did in my down time was.

It was a means of forgetting myself, of giving myself a reason to feel so numb, but it only delayed the progress of my understanding. I don't know if I would have understood myself and my feelings better had I not been drinking, but I would at least have felt healthier. Drinking was simply something I knew how to do, a reflex that I turned to when I was too much in shock to do anything else.

Looking back now, I see that I was in shock for at least a year. I wasn't really sure how I was feeling or what I should be feeling, or if there even could be a normative idea about how grief would progress. I tracked my progress against the popular timelines of grief and felt like they somehow didn't apply to me. I couldn't see acceptance on my horizon and I was deeply troubled when people said grief never really leaves you. I couldn't go on *like that* forever, fearing sleep because of the nightmares that would come, knowing that I would wake and grieve all over again when reality dawned with the morning sun. I had to know it could get better.

It was a consultant in A&E who convinced me of that. He too

had lost a brother in his twenties and he was the only person to reassure me that I would feel happy again. He said he knew how dark the first months of grief could be and that although the scars might never heal, the pain would weaken and my life would return to something manageable. I have realised since that happiness can return, but it does not take grief's place because grief is, in some form or another, forever.

The 'stages of grief' model, which was originally designed to describe the process by which terminally ill people come to understand the end of their lives, has been applied to all grief and all those who grieve. It defines the final stage of grief as acceptance but many experts see this as too clear a full stop. Acceptance is something we can reach, but it doesn't end grief or guarantee that on some days we will not still be depressed by it and find it hard to accept once again. Models built on stages are useful descriptors, but our complex, ever-changing human minds have a tendency to exist outside of easy categorisation. Acceptance was a stage of my grief that I experienced much later but it isn't one that I experience every day.

At the end of the summer after Llŷr's death, I started taking antidepressants. They helped me through that dark time, allowed me to function and to engage with the aspects of my life that I was ignoring in my depression, but I had a sense that they couldn't be an enduring solution. I turned to them in part to numb my pain, in the same way I was numbing myself with alcohol and work, but I knew that I would have to confront my grief and the pain that preceded it. I needed to develop my own resources for coping and finding joy in life, and I needed to build community and support networks.

I struggled to do that, and still do now, which means that I have often had to navigate my return to normality alone. I had support from people close to me at the time but I learned that a lot of people don't know how to engage with the pain of suicide, and particularly that of the young. I think it frightens people, that we lack the culture or the words to shed light on something so dark, and this can mean that those of us who have lost someone in such a way remain somewhat isolated. So it was on my own that I did most of my growth. Death, like life, teaches us a lot of hard lessons, and I learned a lot about grief and happiness in the years after Llŷr's loss. I realised quite how strong and resilient I can be. The best thing that can happen when the worst thing happens is that you realise you can endure almost anything. If that is all that I took from my experience of grief, it would be a powerful lesson, but it was only the first of my insights.

I learned to accept that life is short and not something to be afraid of. The pain of realising that Llŷr's memory will someday be lost, in two or three generations, soon became a point of empowerment for me. I realised that the things I worried about, my reputation or my failures, would not go beyond my lifetime. I would be forgotten and I could take strength in remembering that. So I resolved not to be constrained by my fears and to know that we have a short time in which to connect with others on this earth. I didn't so much resolve to live every day to the fullest, but to remember that everything is temporary: success or failure, pain and joy – they are all moments to be experienced as well as moments that will pass.

That temporary nature of our existence, and the striking

ability of the world to keep on turning regardless of what we do, dawns on me on Llŷr's anniversary each year. I look back to that day and find comfort in the brutal reality that the world simply goes on, whatever we do. A few days after he died, I walked on the beach with my friend Mark. The waves still crashed and the sand was still soft. Kids were still playing and building sandcastles. My brother had killed himself and the sun still shone. In my family's darkest moment, there was probably a house a few doors down filled with laughter. On the worst day of my life, somebody, somewhere, was having the best day of theirs and there is comfort in that. The world does not stop, and it does not watch you or wait for you. So many of us live in fear of what the world thinks of us, but we need not because it always goes on. I have lived through the worst-case scenario and life continues.

I often turn to the worst-case scenario, but at least I try do do so in a far healthier way than I once did. Whereas I used to be preoccupied with how bad things could be, now I ask myself, how bad can anything really be? We may spend our lives in fear of the worst happening but so often that worst-case scenario is genuinely insignificant. Say I am anxious about an upcoming talk – what is the worst that can happen? Maybe I will fumble my words and convey nothing over the course of an hour. Maybe I'll trip and fall as I approach the lectern. Maybe every person in that room will leave thinking less of me. That is the *worst* that can happen, and yet my world will go on. The world will go on. It may be a bad day for me but it may be a great day for someone else, so there is no use becoming preoccupied with it.

These thoughts can lead to greater compassion too. The awareness that your worst day can be someone's best reminds you that the reverse can occur. On my good days, anyone, anywhere, could be going through something terrible. The man who cuts me off at the junction could be rushing to his parents' side because he has lost a brother; the online troll who seems dedicated to making others' lives miserable may be on a journey through grief. The people I once saw as an annoyance are now sketched with the darkness and light of experience. Their actions may be wrong but I have more room for compassion because I now know the reality of invisible pain. That has been a powerful lesson.

My challenges have not completely transformed me, though. We tend to think that people who have been through suffering become noble stoics, able to see the world with admirable perspective, but I still make many of the same mistakes I always did. I still get frustrated and sometimes dwell on things that don't matter, but I prefer to see the positive in that. In the early days of my grief, I sometimes wondered how anything could ever seem important again, given the scale of the experience I had just had, so even my petty frustrations are something to appreciate.

I try to take as many positives from my experience as possible, and although grief may not have taught me total patience or brought me peace, it has made me appreciate what is important in life. I value my life more and the people within it, and I know more than ever how easily they can be lost. If you have someone in your life who you love, remember that someday you will both pass and any troubles you may have will too, so don't dwell on them and try to resolve any disputes you have. Anger is almost always a wasted emotion and conflict is energy that seeks no resolution, so try to find peace with those you care about because nothing and no one is forever.

A lot of these sentiments were summed up by the Latin phrase *memento mori*, which means 'remember you must die'. There is so much wisdom packed into those two small words – that we should not take life too seriously and also that we should not take it for granted, that we should be conscious of death and that we should also value life.

In this country, we shy away from the knowledge that we will die and the reality that people do every day. Our culture is such that we don't speak about death or grief very openly, and, as a result, we fail to support grieving people. I have friends from other cultures who have been shocked by the muted nature of English grief: it is not public, it is not encouraged and the emotion associated with it is something to be hidden. In part, this stems from our Victorian tendency towards suffering in silence. We treat public displays of sadness as something to be ashamed of, when really they are calls to community and requests for support that we would all make if we lived without shame. We are often afraid to engage people we care about in conversations about grief because we worry that we are putting them in a compromising position where they may show their emotions, but one that leaves us with no outlet. The simple fact is that we will all die, and we will all grieve, and there is nothing to be ashamed of, so we must normalise the discussion of life and death in Britain.

I know there is a desire to discuss grief and trauma in this country because when I post about my experiences, there is a deluge of sentiment and connection from people on my channels. My efforts to speak about youth suicide and grief is out of the ordinary because our culture has made silence the norm, but it is only people like you and me who can change that. We must face death and speak to our children about it. We must avoid the superficial stoicism of silence and secrecy and celebrate publicly the people we have lost. We should have more memorials, celebrate more anniversaries and talk about the lives of people who we have lost. Most people who speak to me about Llŷr ask about what it was like to lose him, but I would love to talk about things he loved. Who he was and who he would be now. He would have adored the dogs that my parents got after he passed; he would have loved seeing Lewis Hamilton winning at Silverstone and watching the NBA finals. He would have enjoyed the summer days on which we now remember him. For his sake, and for the sake of those of us who love him, we should not hide from the wonder of his life or the reality of his death.

We shouldn't hide from the conditions that left his sadness untreated either. Some of those measures to create a culture of openness around death and grief would also make space for people to speak openly about their mental health in life. If we are to stop losing people to suicide, we need to continue destigmatising conversations about mental health and start teaching our children to be mentally fit as well as physically fit and academically successful. I would like to see dedicated mental health support teams in every school – something that the British government should be prioritising – and

a clear path for young people to follow when they begin to struggle.
If our environment is not conducive to a young person's wellbeing,
then at least it needs to be conducive to them communicating how
they feel, so that we can make sure that resources are available to
support them through their hardship.

Just as flowers grow upon cemetery plots, I wanted Llŷr's death
to bring good into the world. It was in his name that I dedicated
myself to creating better resources for young people experiencing
mental health challenges. The approach we decided on was Early
Intervention Hubs: community spaces that young people can walk
into at any time to access dedicated mental health support without
engaging the emergency services or sitting on NHS waiting lists.
They will be staffed by young people who are committed to helping
their peers and those a few years younger than them. They will
offer counselling, community and activity, and our intention is
to provide people with the knowledge and support they need to
overcome bouts of depression or mental illness, and realise that they
will be able to do so again in the future. This could impact many
people across many lifetimes and normalise a community-centred
approach to mental health support, rather than one that takes place
in hospitals, institutions and prisons.

Most people who suffer from mental health problems do so
before they are twenty-five, but it can take years or even decades
for them to receive the proper diagnosis. This makes it imperative
that we offer people access to support earlier and more proactively.
Often, people lack the resources or support networks they need
to take care of themselves as young adults, and as a society, we

have a duty to provide them with those things. Moreover, if we can establish connections with people when they are young, we will be able to provide them with support throughout their later lives, and ensure that they make it into their old age.

The Centre for Mental Health estimates that mental ill health costs our country almost £300 billion a year, which is more than the entire budget of the NHS for the same period. It's clear from my experience that a lack of mental health support is at the heart of our overcrowded A&E departments and underperforming workplaces. Making positive, decisive interventions in the mental health and wellbeing of our country could be a social and economic gamechanger.

We need to change our norms around silence. The silence that many people feel they must keep when their mental health suffers. The silence that these people hear when they are brave enough to reach out for help because our public services are too busy dealing with 'the sick' to find time to support those who are growing mentally unwell. The silence that our culture allows to exist around grief and the grieving.

The experience of poor mental health may differ from other life-threatening illnesses because it starts and ends with words, whereas other cases can be described through charts and numbers that cannot be ignored. We need to change this idea of ours. We must listen to people who struggle with their mental health in the very same way we would to someone describing the first symptoms of a potentially fatal physical illness. We must see the lack of mental health provisions in the same stark terms we see a lack of hospital beds or oncologists. The fact that a form of illness exists in the mind does not mean it's less pressing than those existing solely in the body.

Our sense of the mind and the body as two separate entities is a norm that has tripped up generations. The health and wellbeing of our bodies is a crucial driver of the health of our minds, and illnesses of the mind are illnesses of our bodies. As I mentioned earlier, we have normalised 'dualism', a separation of ourselves into two spheres that allows us to treat our minds and bodies in different ways, with a different lack of respect depending on the situation. As much as possible, we should reunite our brains with the bodies they exist in, that they are an inseparable part of. Only then will we be able to focus on creating the conditions that lead to healthy bodies *and* minds.

We need to fuel our bodies and our minds with natural food, we need to move our bodies and our minds through the natural world, and we need to offer our minds and bodies opportunities to relax. We cannot care for one without caring for the other and we cannot continue treating the sicknesses that they develop as part of different universes.

Finally, we cannot continue to treat the grieving as outcasts or lonely people on a necessary procession through simple stages of grief. We will *all* experience grief: almost all of us already have. Our norm is to treat grief as the exception in life but it is in fact the rule. We should all ask ourselves what we would want from our community while we grieved and seek out those who are now grieving to offer it. Life is an incredible thing, in large part because it is finite and because we will all die. We cannot truly live unless we appreciate the reality of death, of dying and of grieving.

If we can do these things – bring an understanding of death into our appreciation of life, treat mental illness with the gravity with which we treat physical illness and commit to living in ways that nourish both our bodies and our minds – we will all be happier and healthier.

We may also save the life of a boy like my brother. I sincerely hope that in some small way Llŷr's loss can teach more people how to care for themselves and care for one another. To value our bodies and minds, to heal sickness and to find health.

9

SO HOW MUCH DO YOU DRINK?

On 4 December 2022, I made the choice to stop drinking. Sitting in that barber's chair while he made friendly conversation, I looked at myself and despaired. I was slowly dying. My eyes looked glassy, my skin sagged and my weight had ballooned to 21 stone. I felt a soreness in my chest that was not only a product of grief but of poor health. I saw the man in the mirror and realised that I had to make a change.

At first, it wasn't clear what that change should be. As I disappeared and reappeared in the mirror behind my barber's hands, I wondered what I could do. I was sick and I was grieving, and in my grief, I had made a pact with my remaining family members that we would stick around for one another, whatever it took. When my fringe was half its previous length and numerous questions had been idly answered, I decided upon the change I needed to make. First, I had to stop drinking.

I had been drinking for fifteen years or so and it was the most normal thing in the world. It was as if I had unwittingly been enrolled in a club of regular drinkers as a teenager and at no point had I or anyone else asked if it was best I remain a member. It was the obvious thing to change, but in some ways, my life and our society had obscured that. The health challenges I was experiencing and the ways in which I was numbing my grief were all inextricably linked to the over-consumption of alcohol. People who study the human body and the human mind could have told me that in minutes, and as someone who has tried to do both, I was aware on some level that the single greatest lever I could pull to protect my health and longevity was sobriety.

It may sound as if I am overplaying the extent of the problem I faced, and the condition of the man I saw in that mirror, but I promise I am not. I knew, as a doctor and as the person who lived inside my sick body, that I was unlikely to make it to forty in the state I was in. My chart would have read: *'thirty-year-old male, obese, struggling with a stressful job and acute grief, problematic relationship with alcohol'*. If I was my own doctor, I would have advised me to make significant lifestyle changes, and if I was my own friend, I would have told me how worried I was. So things had to change but for some reason it was not a duty to myself or my own health that motivated me, but to my family. We had made a solemn promise, the sort of promise that is binding for being forged in the fires of grief, to live on for one another. I was breaking that promise, in some slow way, by ignoring my health. I was dying slowly and I was doing it to myself, which, in the context of the suicide that had precipitated our promise and my own self-destruction, was deeply relevant. I could choose life, in a way we all felt Llŷr had not. I could break the chain of grief and realised that it was only by breaking up with alcohol that I could do so.

And it was a break-up. My relationship with alcohol had lasted longer than any romantic or professional relationship I've ever had. I had been a drinker before I had been a good student or doctor, before I had known love or loss. Alcohol had been my reward system and my anxiety medication before I had really worked for anything or faced true struggles. I'd been introduced to it as a young teenager, handed a potentially destructive substance that ruins millions of lives worldwide and told *learn to control this*, as if that was a normal gift for a society to bestow. Moreover, I was taught in time that if I could not control it, *I* had a problem. It was not the society that gave a teenager a drug, while celebrating it at every sports match and concert, and using it to signify victory and commiseration. I, the individual, was to take this potential poison and be told it was a good thing, but if it became bad then that was a sign of my weakness.

So I drank through my teenage years to manage my social anxiety. The boy who went from being a social outcast to a semi-accepted member of the cool kids did so with a beer in hand to ease his worries. It made me less afraid to attend the parties I would otherwise have avoided and to speak to the people who had once ostracised me. If I had too much of it, I was a party animal, or a lad, and if I had ever questioned whether it was actually worth having, I would have been considered abnormal.

In fact, I was odd in some ways, or at least different, and knowing that would have helped me understand my relationship to booze. I was a neurodivergent person and the reality is that people on the autistic and ADHD spectrum face particular challenges with substance misuse. Some studies estimate that a quarter of people being treated for alcohol and substance abuse have ADHD, and that there is also a far greater likelihood of young people with ADHD using alcohol than their neurotypical peers. So I was part of a group that regularly faces challenges with alcohol misuse, and often has difficulties managing impulses and addictive, dopamine-seeking behaviours. I was also introduced to alcohol before I'd had a chance to learn that.

People with ADHD are more likely to be drawn in by alcohol and to develop dangerous impulse-driven relationships with it, but we are also prone to appreciate its potential value as a depressant. Alcohol, as defined by the World Health Organization (WHO), contains the psychoactive toxin ethanol, which apart from killing around 2.5 million people a year also acts as a depressant that reduces the quality of life for many more. This means that it slows down your brain functioning and neural activity by depressing your central nervous system. To a person with ADHD, this can be an incredibly attractive proposition. An overactive mind is drawn to this effect, and to a naive and impulsive teenager, it can offer both short-term relief and a pathway to despair.

For a young person like me to be given access to alcohol before being given access to therapy or someone who could diagnose my neurodiversity seems like a recipe for disaster, but that is a norm in British culture. We treat the over-consumption of alcohol as a rite of passage, something that marks the transition to adulthood. We offer very little dedicated support or advice to teenagers on the realities and risks of alcohol consumption, while assuming they will behave like all generations before them. Some will sink into substance misuse and some will swim. Many will develop a harmful relationship with alcohol, but many others will become 'normal' members of society who drink at the 'correct' times – evenings, weekends, sunny days and sports events, when there is something to celebrate and when there is something to commiserate.

I didn't develop an addiction but I had a problematic relationship with alcohol from my very first drink. I drank as a teenager to manage my social anxiety, to self-medicate and self-administer a drug in place of a therapeutic or medical intervention. I continued to do so at university. Just as we graduate from secondary to higher education, so too do many people in Britain move up in terms of their alcohol consumption. I went out more and I drank more, but I grew no better at managing my social anxiety without alchohol. Why would I? We seem to accept that university is a time for excess, a place where alcohol is celebrated, and there is very little recognition of how this could present problems for young people. This can be an incredibly fun experience, but we set a dangerous precedent when we give young adults their first taste of independence and assume they want to do so surrounded by alcohol. University offers us a chance to learn the habits and mindsets that we will carry with us into our adult lives, to learn who we are for the life that follows.

What followed for me was a highly stressful profession, and I worked on the assumption that good weeks were for celebrating at the pub and hard ones were for decompressing in the very same place. I had embedded drinking habits and although I managed my relationship with alcohol, I still relied on it. Alcohol was a way to cope with my workplace stress but it was also something that stopped me from recovering from it effectively. I would spend Friday and Saturday nights at the pub, and return to the high-octane A&E department on a Monday. This meant that my life was spent working, drinking or recovering. Where was the living?

The regularity of drinking was never my great problem, but the amount I would consume when I did drink was. My lack of impulse control made me a classic binge drinker. People would assume that because I didn't drink every day, I didn't really have a problem, but I think this reflects more about our society than it does about me. I may not have been physically addicted to alcohol but I certainly had a problem with it. I used alcohol to make my life more bearable. It helped me avoid social anxiety and distract myself from burnout, and it took me away from myself and the processing that I needed to do. Alcohol was a crutch that stopped me from growing resilient, from learning self-care and from being comfortable to sit with myself.

Drinking was a prerequisite for having a good time and that meant I never really learned what 'good times' meant to me. It was only when I started relying on it to help me through a bad time that I saw how deep my dependency went. It was one thing to need alcohol to enjoy life but another entirely to use it for avoiding sadness. It was in my grief when I finally realised that. I knew I had been drinking more since Llŷr's death. The hole in my heart and my life that opened up with his loss was there to be filled, and I did that with food and drink. On some level, I believed that those things could push my sadness away, but in the barber's chair I saw that there was a price to pay for my distraction. It would be my destruction and I had to act on it for my family's sake.

So I stopped. I left the barber's and walked out into a grey London afternoon, but it was what I didn't do then that changed me. I didn't go to the pub or message the drinking buddies I had collected. In fact, I didn't do much at all. I was at a loss. What do people do when they are not working and not drinking? I had no idea. In part that is because I had never explored sober hobbies, but also because British culture makes very little space for activities that don't involve a few pints. Alcohol is such a part of the social fabric of this country that I felt like an outcast on the day I made the best decision of my life.

You might be surprised to find out that was the hardest aspect of my newfound sobriety. I did not struggle with serious cravings or withdrawals, but I felt entirely aimless without alcohol. It had framed my life in such a way that I did not know who I was or what to do without it. Where did I go in my down-time, how would I meet my friends or make new ones, what even *was* a Saturday night? The answers to those questions were not immediately clear and it took some time before I was able to find better ways to use my time.

The first step towards finding purpose was deciding that I would make my health a priority. It made sense – I had stopped drinking because I was worried about my health but, moreover, it gave me something to work at. It was not enough to remove something from

my life; I had to add something. So I added endorphins in place
of toxins and the connection of group exercise rather than the
fraternity of the bar stool.

The endorphins were a fantastic substitute, far more satisfying
than alcohol and accessible without the trade-off of a hangover. Re-
creating social connections was harder to do. I joined exercise classes
and started going to running groups, but my social anxiety stopped
me from seeing them as places where I could make friends. I had to
learn to speak to people in my natural state and I really struggled.
I felt odd trying to start a friendly chat with someone at Barry's Boot
Camp or a run club as I lacked the confidence to do so. My sense of
social norms was that conversations could be started in a pub but
not at a workout, that the very healthy practice of building human
connections was only normal when allied to the unhealthy practice
of drinking.

I see now that this was both my problem and a problem with the
society in which I had learned my logic, but it took time for me to
understand this and adapt. This was hard – but hard things often
prove to be satisfying. Learning that I could socialise without a
drink and questioning things that I had taken for granted gave me
a sense of progress and self-efficacy. I had taken dependency and
questionable social norms for granted, and while undoing this was
a struggle, it was one which gave me a sense of pride.

I had to adapt to the new structure of my weeks. I couldn't
work on the assumption that Friday and Saturday nights were
for drinking, and weekend days for recovering, so something
had to change. Often, that meant spending Friday and Saturday

nights alone, and in time, I grew more comfortable with that. I started to question the idea that weekend evenings are somehow special (due to our five-day working week) and once I realised that early mornings could be just as fun as late nights, I started to feel more at ease with my new schedule. I may have lost the idea of Saturday night that I'd once had but I had gained a new appreciation of Sunday mornings. I learned, as many sober people do, that we can gain new meaning in sobriety even if the transition is hard.

This transition would be easier if our cultural norms progressed in a few small ways. The first would be in the normalisation of social activities outside of pubs, clubs and bars. I would love to meet people on a Saturday night to play chess or attend a book club, and I'd love to play sports late into the night or go on dates in places that are not based around booze. I don't think that alcohol has to be off the table in any of these spaces but I just think that a lot of people would feel more enfranchised if alcohol wasn't the establishment's defining purpose. A non-drinker in a pub can feel like an odd one out, it's like going to a restaurant when you're not hungry, but I think spaces with a focus on something other than alcohol would really change that. Non-drinkers would also be saved from the sense that other people are somehow put out by our sobriety, as if our choice not to drink somehow suggests their choices are inherently problematic. I noticed this more in pubs than anywhere else. For instance, no one notices if you have a diet coke at the theatre or cinema, but in a pub, it feels to many people as if you are breaking the social contract.

I don't think this necessarily means fewer people at pubs and bars, but maybe more of a continental attitude to their purpose.

I think my move to sobriety was helped immeasurably by the introduction of a dedicated fitness regime into my life. It is very difficult to take something away from your life without adding something else to replace it, and that is how I approached my fitness routine. I substituted evenings for mornings and pints for Pilates (OK, maybe not Pilates – but it does look fun). After I got over my initial social anxiety, I realised that fitness and wellness spaces are actually fantastic places to meet people and share in a communal experience. The added benefit was that every drink I didn't have made a positive impact on my fitness: I was getting fitter by exercising but also by not consuming alcohol.

I don't know how I would have felt about sobriety without the endorphins and psychological release of exercise. I found that without alcohol I was suddenly left to confront and process a lot of sadness and a great deal of trauma that I had ignored, and it really helped to have activities which made my mind feel clearer and my body relaxed. I never expected that giving up alcohol would open me up to this new challenge. I had expected it to involve a physical withdrawal and possibly a social one, but I never realised that I would be withdrawing from such a potent defence (or deference) mechanism. In fact, the strength of feeling that I uncovered in sobriety is a testament to how successfully I had sublimated my sadness with alcohol. My grief rushed in, unmediated, every night and every morning. My anxiety about the future, my work and my social life could no longer be numbed.

I thought I had made the decision to give up alcohol but, in truth, I had made a decision to meet myself and accept all the difficulty that came with that.

It may surprise you to learn that this was particularly pronounced when I slept and when I woke up each morning. Most of us understand that alcohol impacts the quality of our sleep and assume that sobriety must immediately yield restful nights, but in the short term I experienced the opposite. First, it can take many months for our brains and our sleep patterns to recover from repeated alcohol use. For me, the hardest period of that recovery was in the first two weeks, when, left without sedative effect of alcohol, I would struggle to relax and experience a deep, full sleep. Without sedation, a newly sober brain can be hyperactive. More importantly, though, the nightmares that I had drunk away for a number of years were now free to enter and the floodgates opened. I struggled terribly with painful dreams and restless waking because my body was adapting to 'normal' patterns of deep and REM sleep, which results in more frequent and vivid dreams. It felt as if all of the trauma I had put aside had somehow accrued interest. I still knew that sobriety was what I needed to do, though. On some level, my decision in the barber's chair was a recognition that I could not sit upon my pain any longer and that only left me with the option of engaging it, however hard that was.

It did get better. After about ten weeks my mind had adapted to the new normal of sleep. By then, I was able to approach my pain through therapy, empowered by a good rest and the sense of self-assurance that only comes with choosing to do something hard for good reasons. I was proud of myself, and my resilience, and that both strengthened my mind and made me feel capable of strengthening it further. I also saw my body change rapidly. In the course of a year, I lost seven stone. The puffiness in my face reduced over a few weeks, my eyes got brighter and whiter and the acne I had struggled with for years disappeared. People told me I looked ten years younger. I couldn't put a number on it but I felt like *myself*. I still sometimes felt uncertain, anxious and afraid, but I was closer to those feelings than I had ever been, embracing the difficulty of facing them head on rather than exhausting myself trying to run away.

A short while into my sobriety journey, I went to see a cardiologist. I had been experiencing chest pains on exertion and was pretty worried. Thankfully after a full check up and tests on my heart, everything seemed to be OK. His view had been that if my previous lifestyle had continued, I would in time have damaged my cardiovascular system in quite a significant way. He told me that my lifestyle changes were sure to have a positive effect on my broader health and my cardiovascular system in particular, that I had made those changes at a good time – but that, regardless, it would never be too late. I must say that the conversation felt like a stark reminder of why I could never go back.

I think the ability of the human body to repair itself is something we should all take encouragement from. Most self-imposed health challenges can be mitigated if we make a concerted effort to improve our lifestyle. It can certainly be hard. Sobriety and weight loss are notoriously difficult to maintain, but they are not impossible, and if we can commit to ourselves and to saving our own bodies then we are on the right track. I had to learn to value myself, and my own life, and only by realising that I was worth preserving did I start to take the steps necessary to save myself. Along the way, I have discovered that doing something for my body has been a great help to my mind.

I wonder whether an increased understanding of mental and physical health, and the interconnections between the two, lies at the root of the changing patterns of alcohol consumption in younger generations. People born after the year 2000 are far less likely to drink alcohol than any generation before them (around 39 per cent of them do not drink at all, according to a 2024 YouGov poll), and they are also notably much more aware of how to improve their mental and physical health than their forebears. I think there must be some link between these two facts, but it may only be one of the reasons why youth alcohol consumption in the UK is declining so markedly.

Young people I have spoken to on the subject seem to have progressed to the realisations that I have without experiencing the harms of prolonged alcohol use first. Many believe alcohol consumption to be unattractive due to its expense, physical risks and emotional impacts. I find it particularly interesting that many of them use language that has so often characterised youthful rebellion to describe their decisions. Like the hippies a few generations before them, they question the value of working long hours to *earn* a weekend, but they also ask why the weekend they would choose to earn would be spent dissociating with alcohol. They look at their parents' generation and ask themselves whether this is the life that they want for themselves – working hard just to spend their evenings and weekends at the pub or drinking at home. Things are changing, and for many young people, drinking is simply an expensive, messy hobby that they would rather relegate from its status as the primary form of social engagement.

This is laudable and a reflection of the strength of character that new generations must display to displace old habits. Young people are bombarded with alcohol advertising in the same ways the rest of us are, but they seem to have developed the media literacy to separate marketing from reality. Maybe they sense how odd it is that every sports tournament is sponsored by booze brands or that a sunny afternoon in the park cannot just be a sunny afternoon in the park, but has to be 'Pimm's o'clock'. My generation may not have sensed the awkward association of elite athletes with lager or F1 drivers with Champagne, but if that consciousness has developed in the newer generation, it will be hard to shift.

The least we can do as a society is to encourage more spaces for sober-curious young people to socialise in a new way. Much of this enterprise will be dictated by market forces, as new businesses will open to serve this demographic, but we cannot just leave this to chance. I think this risks alcohol's loss becoming exclusively social media and online gaming's gain. A move away from alcohol consumption should not entail a move towards isolation, and I think that policymakers should work to make it easier for new business owners to open social spaces that are not built around booze. I believe that the logic behind our Early Support Hubs, that healthy dedicated spaces for young people can be transformative, can be extended from those who are at risk of mental health challenges to those who are simply trying to find new ways to flourish. Community arts spaces, sports facilities, places to dance, read and play can all become parts of a healthier society that prioritises social connection over inebriation. If we can create these spaces and glorify these good things in our media rather than alcohol, we can celebrate a new kind of healthy hedonism that doesn't rely on drinking.

I can say with a great degree of certainty that this would be music to the ears of my colleagues in A&E. We rarely had to treat reading-related injuries or people who got hurt from the overconsumption of art. What we did do was spend every Friday and Saturday night stretched to breaking point, picking up the pieces of Britain's problematic relationship with alcohol. If that can change, if moderation and sobriety become normalised and we can diversify our ways of socialising, then we could have a healthier, happier country and an NHS that is free to treat people who are sick. The only group who might be impacted by such a change would be the multibillion-pound alcohol industry, but even they could benefit from a less alcohol-dependent culture. The low– and no-alcohol market was worth around £380 million at the end of 2024 and is forecast to grow to as much as £800 million by 2028. So there is potential for these companies to continue profitably without contributing to tens of thousands of alcohol-related deaths each year.

The writer Johann Hari, who I spoke to on my podcast, once said that 'the opposite of addiction is not sobriety, it is human connection'. I think our culture has been addicted to alcohol for a long time and in part this has endured because we believe that alcohol is a prerequisite for connection. We all have a natural impulse to spend time with other people, sharing in something and being disinhibited. Alcohol is one way to do this, but it is not the best way, and it is certainly not the only way. If we can find greater human connection, we can reduce our culture's addiction to alcohol. We do not need to give it up entirely, although for some people like me that may be necessary, but we could start to create connections and see where we end up.

If I look back at my discussion of our very British attitude to grief, which requires sublimating emotions and bottling up sentiment until we are fit to burst, I can't help but see a connection to our alcohol culture. We are so inhibited that we struggle to speak to one another without a pint. The men in my community would never dream of letting each other know that they care for one other but would readily put their best friend to bed after a big night out. We struggle to tell each other when we are at a low, but we might finally let our nearest and dearest know that we are struggling should we become very drunk. Alcohol may not be the reason Britain is repressed but relying on a dangerous substance to open up means that we avoid engaging with the root causes. We should try getting close to one another, sharing our feelings, and experiencing fraternity and community without booze. We might just find we are healthier and happier for it.

I lost my brother to suicide and in response, I almost lost myself to alcohol. I hope that our culture can take a long, hard look at itself in the mirror, as I once did. If we do not like what we see, we should make a change to what we call normal because we should not need to numb ourselves to the world. It may be filled with pain but it is also filled with deep, profound beauty. Pain may be hard to process, and it may sometimes be hard to endure, but we should not force ourselves to forget.

We must foster connections to one another and the world around us, and normalise doing so without a drink in our hand.

10

AM I NORMAL?

This question has preoccupied me a lot in my adult life. Answering it has required me to both understand myself and the world that has formed me, to see the good in both and the opportunities. I'm grateful that I'm now at a point where I feel well-placed to answer it, even if the answer is not entirely simple.

My response to the question 'Am I normal?' is both yes and no. There is a simple answer and there is a complex one. The simple answer is, of course, that I am not normal. If I approach my mind purely through an ADHD lens, then I am the definition of difference. The opposite of a typical mind is a neurodivergent one and I am proud to say that I am abnormal. In my eyes, this abnormality is neither a good nor a bad thing. Disability campaigners often point out that it is our world that is disabling, that their bodies and minds would be perfectly able if the world did not disable them through its design. I believe this to be true and relevant in the context of my normality and my ADHD (whether or not that is even considered a disability). When we speak about normality, we often think we are talking about what is right or what is good, when in fact we are talking about what is accounted for: my mind may not be normal but that is only a problem if it exists in systems that don't have the resources or approaches to account for its divergence.

Let's begin with education, as it's the first point at which difference is problematised and a key example of how a narrow understanding of normality can create broad problems for people across our society. Neurodivergent children, and particularly those with ADHD, are often caught in the 'problematic provision loop'. Children as young as four can be characterised as 'problems' if they struggle to cope at school in terms of their attainment, attendance and behaviour. These negative experiences lead to higher drop-out rates and an internalised belief that they are problematic people.

Now let's consider the fact that people with ADHD are massively overrepresented in the criminal justice system. A significant proportion of people in prison will have been 'problematised' in childhood, when reflections of neurodivergence were treated as unruliness or naughtiness. We see here that misdiagnosing these young people's differences as problems will in some cases have placed them at odds with the people that care for them, playing no small part in their later route to imprisonment. We would all benefit from disrupting this 'education to prison pipeline', as better education and crime reduction could go hand in hand. Given that some studies estimate that around a quarter of the prison population has ADHD, it's worthwhile to ask how better provisions for such pupils in schools could reduce harm.

Which speaks to how I think we should approach the question 'Am I normal?' – and the fact that it is meaningless unless allied to the question 'Am I a problem?' In my view, there is no cost to an individual or a society from a person being different unless that individual's difference is made a problem by society. I was fortunate to meet people who saw me beyond the problem that I appeared to present and who gave me opportunities to flourish. When we ask whether we are normal, we should be asking whether we are flourishing, and we need to change how we design our society if we are going to discover a positive answer to that question.

Remember the bell curve I talked about at the start of this book? (See page 4.) Those people, the 'absolute normal' (or median and mode – welcome back to GCSE maths), only account for a small portion of society, so we should not build our provisions entirely around them, as their perfect normality is actually abnormal when we look at the whole set.

So who do we build society for, then? I think we currently design our provisions around a broader subsection, which maybe covers 80 per cent of the graph, 40 per cent on either side of that perfect middle. What we are left with is 10 per cent at either extreme for whom we don't account. Because there is a far smaller number of people in the bottom and top 10 per cent of any bell curve, as a society we deem it cheaper and more straightforward (apparently) to discount them from our programme design. I think this is a mistake. If I was to simplify my thinking down to one idea, it is that we would have a far healthier society, from schools to prisons and hospitals to workplaces, if we dedicated more of our time and resources to understanding the needs of those two sets of outliers. Whether we are talking about ADHD, physical disability or wealth, we would cut our costs and generate disproportionate progress if we focused on what is happening in those areas of difference, of abnormality.

Which brings us to the end of my first answer to the question 'Am I normal', which is 'No, and if we saw that as less of a problem, we would all be better off.' That is the easy answer in the sense that I'm starting here with a very clear, singular form of difference – a medical diagnosis of neurodivergence. The complex answer to the question of my normality is more fractured because it encompasses many more things that we have discussed in this book and the very problematic norms that we have all accepted. In society's eyes, I am normal in some ways and in many ways I am not. To be abnormal is to have friction with the society we are in and our response is either to try to change ourselves to fit in or to work to make our society more inclusive. In many ways, I am not normal because I have chosen to do the latter. To repeat a statement I made about myself in the Introduction:

I am not normal because I have chosen to speak publicly about suicide and grief. The normal response to grief, as governed by (British) social norms, is to be quiet about it and in the context of suicide, to be silent. In this case, speaking up and showing vulnerability is abnormal, but it is also crucial if we are to create healthier norms around grief. Therefore, my abnormality is a necessary price to pay for the normalisation of something important. Again, this reflects how normal does not mean right and how abnormality is something to strive for when we want to make a change.

So, I am normal because I have struggled with my dependencies and abnormal because I can admit that fact without shame. If the opposite of addiction is human connection, then honesty about the vulnerabilities we all share is crucial to protect us all from the loneliness and isolation of these harmful habits. No one should live in private shame for the shopping they are compelled to do, the cigarettes they want to smoke or the food they feel they can't stop eating. The compulsion or addiction itself is hard enough, but to have that experience *alone* is far harder.

I am normal because I have felt lonely. I may be an outlier for admitting it to the world. Technology now spreads our connections further and wider than has ever been possible, but it can also spread our interconnection thin. Modern life can be lonesome and it will take a concerted effort by individuals to recreate the communities that serve as an antidote to that loneliness. We have normalised a less interdependent world and I would argue that is unnatural, that in becoming estranged we all feel strange. I hope my willingness to share my vulnerability to isolation encourages you to reach out to someone if you, or they, could benefit from connection. I hope my acceptance of appearing as an outlier stops others from feeling left on the outside.

I am normal because I grieve, but I may be strange for questioning why so many of us are left to grieve alone. There is no shame in feeling the sharp point of a loved one's death but there is shame in how our culture denies our common experience of it. We treat grief as a rare and secret experience that we hope to avoid lest it catches and infects us. Grief is not a virus, it is the most normal of human experiences for beings that live, love and die, and it is only through willingness to admit to our grief and to reach out to others who experience it that we can normalise a culture that supports the grieving. The sting of loss should not be intensified by a call to suffer privately – this was not normal as previous times in history and it is not normal across many cultures in the world. In Britain today, we have a duty to rediscover solidarity in grief.

It should be clear that, most of all, I am abnormal because I am not afraid to admit that I am. I am grateful that I realised the pain that my struggle to fit in was causing as well as the opportunity I had to live more authentically by admitting to my difference. I built a house of cards upon foundations of normality that I neither understood nor needed. I drank to fit in, I grieved silently to avoid standing out and I ate as I was told to by companies who profit off processed foods that would seem strange to every generation of humans who ever came before us. Then I realised that my efforts to twist myself into the shape of society's norms were tying me in knots. I untied myself and found my own form and function. Normal function does not mean doing things the way they have always been done or the way others seem to be doing them, but the ability to move through the world without the friction of inauthenticity. What we're told is normal is not always what is good; our minds and our bodies can tell us that and when we grow anxious or sick, isolated and depressed, this tells us that the norms we are living beneath are causing us friction and pain.

So take pride in abnormality. Seek it and grow into it. If you can, help someone else to be authentically abnormal. If you're an outlier, take pride in it and try to create space for others who sit at the edges of society's bell curve. This could be a grand project of modernity. Just as our ancestors broadened out the scope of who counted in society and moderated its norms to include those on the outside, so too can we push the project of inclusivity forward. Through more inclusive schools, we could reduce the prison population; through more inclusive communities, we might just relieve our overburdened hospitals.

I believe this wholeheartedly because it is only by appreciating our own difference that we can understand how the world could be different. And it's only by imagining what this could look like that that we can understand how it could change for the better. I have spent a great deal of time looking back over my life in the last few years, and although I've come to the conclusion that I am not normal, I have become happier and healthier for understanding how. I believe that if our society goes through a similar process of reflection, we will all be happier and healthier.

This journey, which started as baby steps with Toddla T, has helped me mature into a man who is less afraid of himself and the world. By understanding my past and the world that forms my present, I now appreciate how it could be improved in the future. I may have to accept standing out and appearing different if I am to make the changes I hope to see. You might have to do the same. But if we do it together, we can make our differences normal. Then, we can make the world a better place.

Yours,
Dr Alex George

BIBLIOGRAPHY

Carter, B., Payne, M., Rees, P., Sohn, S. Y., Brown, J., & Kalk, N. J. (2024), 'A Multi-school Study in England, to Assess Problematic Smartphone Usage and Anxiety and Depression', *Acta Paediatrica, International Journal of Paediatrics*, 113(10): 2240–48

Csikszentmihalyi, M. (1990), *Flow: the Psychology of Optimal Experience*, New York: Harper & Row

Foulkes, L. (2024), *Coming of Age: How Adolescence Shapes Us*, London: Vintage

Ginapp, C., Macdonald-Gagnon, G., Angarita, G., Bold, K., Potenza, M., (2022), 'The Lived Experiences of Adults with Attention-Deficit/ Hyperactivity Disorder: A Rapid Review of Qualitative Evidence', *Frontiers in Psychiatry*, Vol. 13

Haidt, J. (2024), *The Anxious Generation: How the Great Rewiring of Childhood Is Causing an Epidemic of Mental Illness*, London: Penguin Press

Hemez, P., Brent, J. J., Mowen, T. J. (2020), 'Exploring the School-to-Prison Pipeline: How School Suspensions Influence Incarceration During Young Adulthood', *Youth Violence and Juvenile Justice*, 18(3):235–55

Liu, C., Townes, P., Panesar, P. et al. (2024), 'Executive Function in ADHD and ASD: A Scoping Review', *Review Journal of Autism and Developmental Disorders*

May, F., Ford, T., Janssens, A., Newlove-Delgado, T., Emma Russell, A., Salim, J., Ukoumunne, O. C., Hayes, R. (2021), 'Attainment, Attendance, and School Difficulties in UK Primary Schoolchildren with Probable ADHD', *British Journal of Educational Psychology*, 91(1):442–62

Mintel (2024), 'Attitudes Towards Low-And-No-Alcohol Drinks UK', *UK Consumer Attitudes Report*

NASUWT (2024), Teachers Wellbeing Survey Report 2024, Birmingham: NASUWT. Available at: https://www.nasuwt.org.uk/static/ 17ad7ef2-879e-40d4-96b3c014e605746a/Teachers-Wellbeing-Survey-Report-2024.pdf

Russell, A. E., Benham-Clarke, S., Ford, T., Eke, H., Price, A., Mitchell, S., Newlove-Delgado, T., Moore, D., Janssens, A. (2023), 'Educational Experiences of Young People with ADHD in the UK: Secondary Analysis of Qualitative Data from the CATCh-uS Mixed-Methods Study', *British Journal of Educational Psychology*

Silva, I., Costa, D. (2023), 'Consequences of Shift Work and Night Work: A Literature Review', *Healthcare, 11*(10), 1410

Torquati, L., Mielke, G. I., Brown, W. J., Burton, N. W., Kolbe-Alexander, T. L. (2019), 'Shift Work and Poor Mental Health: A Meta-Analysis of Longitudinal Studies', *American Journal of Public Health*, 109(11): e13-e20

Twenge, J. M., Campbell, W. K. (2018), 'Associations Between Screen Time and Lower Psychological Well-being Among Children and Adolescents: Evidence from a Population-based Study,' *Preventive Medicine Reports*, 18; 12:271–83

RESOURCES AND FURTHER READING

Organisations

Mind – www.mind.org.uk

ADHD Foundation – www.adhdfoundation.org.uk

ADHD UK – adhduk.co.uk

YoungMinds – www.youngminds.org.uk

The Mix – www.themix.org.uk

Podcasts

ADHD Chatter

Stompcast

Further Reading

Feel-Good Productivity, Ali Abdaal

Atomic Habits, James Clear

And How Does That Make You Feel?, Joshua Fletcher

Coming of Age: How Adolescence Shapes Us, Lucy Foulkes

The Mind Manual, Dr Alex George

The Unexpected Joy of Being Sober, Catherine Gray

The Anxious Generation, Jonathan Haidt

ADHD – Living Without Brakes, Martin L. Kutscher MD

Attached: Are You Anxious, Avoidant or Secure?, Dr Amir Levine and
    Rachel S. F. Heller

Addicted to Anxiety, Owen O'Kane

The Chimp Paradox, Professor Steve Peters

Why Has Nobody Told Me This Before?, Dr Julie Smith

The Power of Now, Eckhart Tolle

INDEX

ACKNOWLEDGEMENTS

This has by far been the most difficult book I've written and yet, at the same time, the most rewarding. Going through my life and looking closely at events and experiences under the microscope has been really hard emotionally. However, this process has allowed me to understand myself better and actually find a great deal of comfort and acceptance. I suppose what I'm trying to say is that it was all worth it.

I have needed a great deal of support in writing this book and have very much leaned on my dear friend Oscar Millar to help bring it all together. Oscar, I am so incredibly grateful for you, both professionally and as a friend throughout all of this.

I must also thank Carly Cook, Harry Grenville and Abby Wagge in particular. You have been incredible, thank you. To Jo Morrell, Katie Forsythe, Alex Stetter and the rest of the fantastic Octopus team, thank you for your expertise and for giving me the opportunity to tell this story. I hope it helps others on their quest for self-acceptance.

Looking back over my life, it's clear to me just how important my friends and family have been. It's been quite the ride so far and I couldn't have done it without you. I am lucky to be loved by some truly wonderful people.

Finally, thank you to you, the reader. The support, love and inspiration I've felt from you over the years has kept me going, even when times have been tough. I appreciate you all.

ABOUT THE AUTHOR

Dr Alex George is a mental health campaigner and educator. A former A&E doctor, he brings a unique perspective from the frontline of healthcare to his mission of improving the nation's mental fitness.

Alex is a leading advocate for early mental health support. He spent four years as the Youth Mental Health Ambassador to the UK government, has worked closely with YoungMinds to provide funding for Mental Health Support Teams in schools and has helped pioneer Early Support Hubs. He uses his *Stompcast* podcast and his social media channels to reach as many people as possible, and has brought important issues to the forefront through his television documentaries, which include *Dr Alex: Our Young Mental Health Crisis* for BBC One and *Alcohol-Free Booze: Is It Worth It?*

He is the author of four *Sunday Times* bestsellers, including *Live Well Every Day*, *The Mind Manual* and *A Better Day*, which won Children's Non-Fiction Book of the Year at the British Book Awards.

Alex believes that no matter where you are at with your mental health right now, there is always hope for a better day.

RAISING READERS
Books Build Bright Futures

Dear Reader,

We'd love your attention for one more page to tell you about the crisis in children's reading, and what we can all do.

Studies have shown that reading for fun is the **single biggest predictor of a child's future life chances** – more than family circumstance, parents' educational background or income. It improves academic results, mental health, wealth, communication skills, ambition and happiness.[1]

The number of children reading for fun is in rapid decline. Young people have a lot of competition for their time. In 2024, 1 in 10 children and young people in the UK aged 5 to 18 did not own a single book at home.[2]

Hachette works extensively with schools, libraries and literacy charities, but here are some ways we can all raise more readers:

- Reading to children for just 10 minutes a day makes a difference
- Don't give up if children aren't regular readers – there will be books for them!
- Visit bookshops and libraries to get recommendations
- Encourage them to listen to audiobooks
- Support school libraries
- Give books as gifts

There's a lot more information about how to encourage children to read on our website: **www.RaisingReaders.co.uk**

Thank you for reading.

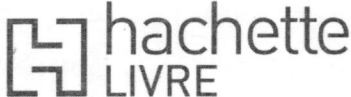

[1] OECD, '21st-Century Readers: Developing Literacy Skills in a Digital World', 2021, https://www.oecd.org/en/publications/21st-century-readers_a83d84cb-en.html

[2] National Literacy Trust, 'Book Ownership in 2024', November 2024, https://literacytrust.org.uk/research-services/research-reports/book-ownership-in-2024